SBL

D0255701

A
ide

7/6/15

li
d

Please return/renew this item by the last date
above. You can renew on-line at
**www.library.lbhf.gov.uk/**
or by phone
**020 8753 2400**

h&f
putting residents first

**Hammersmith & Fulham Libraries**

HAMMERSMITH _FULHAM

3 8005 01338 389 3

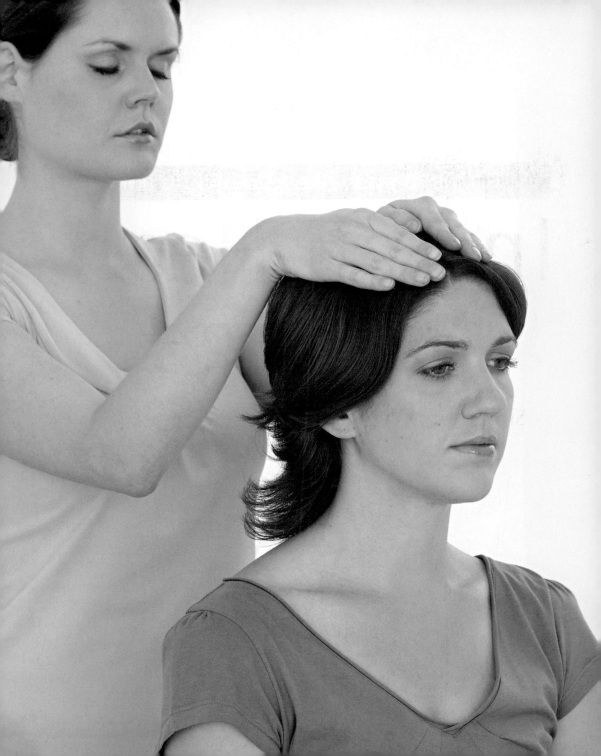

# A Gaia Busy Person's Guide

# Indian Head Massage

## Simple routines for home, work & travel

### Eilean Bentley

*Reconnect with yourself and the planet*

First published in Great Britain in 2007 by Gaia, a division of Octopus Publishing Group Ltd, 2–4 Heron Quays, London E14 4JP

Copyright © Octopus Publishing Group Ltd 2007

Distributed in the United States and Canada by Sterling Publishing Co., Inc, 387 Park Avenue South, New York, NY 10016-8810

All rights reserved. No part of this work may be reproduced or utilized in any form or by any means, electronic or mechanical, including photocopying, recording or by any information storage and retrieval system, without the prior written permission of the publisher.

The right of Eilean Bentley to be identified as the author of this work has been asserted in accordance with section 77(1) of the Copyright, Designs and Patents Act 1988, United Kingdom.

ISBN-13: 978-1-85675-275-6
ISBN-10: 1-85675-275-5

A CIP catalogue record for this book is available from the British Library

Printed and bound in China

10 9 8 7 6 5 4 3 2 1

| London Borough of Hammersmith & Fulham | |
| --- | --- |
| SHE | |
| 3 8005 01338 389 3 | |
| Askews | Jul-2009 |
| H 615.822 | £9.99 |
| 2469415 | |

**DISCLAIMER**

*Massage should not be considered as a replacement for professional medical treatment: a physician should be consulted in all matters relating to health and especially in relation to any symptoms that may require diagnosis or medical attention. While the advice and information in this book are believed to be accurate, neither the author nor the publisher can accept any legal responsibility for any injury sustained while following any of the suggestions made herein.*

# Contents

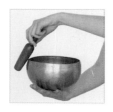 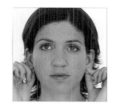 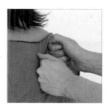 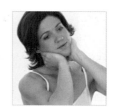

# Introduction

As part of the ancient holistic tradition of Ayurvedic healing, Indian head massage has many benefits for both physical and mental health. The relief of stress alone can alleviate many symptoms such as headaches, high blood pressure, muscle aches, indigestion, dependence on substances like drugs or alcohol, irritable bowel syndrome, irrational fears and tempers, anger, depression, lack of confidence, poor concentration, and anxiety.

## BANISH THE NEGATIVE

When the muscles in your head, neck, shoulders, and upper back are relaxed, negative feelings such as anxiety, fear, and anger are released. Your mind will feel more harmonious and in tune with everything around you, helping you to be more creative, clear, and focused. When mental tiredness and a general lack of energy disappear, your enthusiasm for life bursts forth. At the same time, your inner calm can also infect others, allowing relationships to become more co-operative and easy to manage.

## FREE UP THE PHYSICAL

Together with meditation, visualization, and breathing exercises (see pages 10 and 12–13), Indian head massage encourages correct, deep abdominal breathing and whole-body muscle relaxation. This in turn improves blood and lymph circulation, helping cells to receive a good supply of oxygen and other nutrients.

Massaging your upper back, shoulders, forehead, and eyebrows relieves the tension that can cause

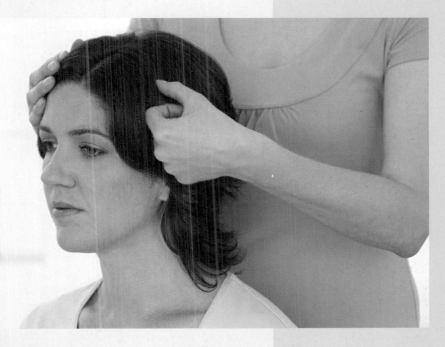

tiredness and strain within the muscles of your eyes. Relaxing and stretching the muscles of your neck and shoulders will help to release toxins from your brain, skin, and other tissues. Massage will also ease stiffness from neck and shoulder joints, aiding flexibility and movement. And, of course, the improved circulation within your scalp helps to enhance the condition, strength, and regrowth of your hair. (In India, gentle massage is even thought to help stimulate growth hormones and brain development in babies and young children.)

All in all, head massage is a wonderful all-round therapy that will leave you feeling revitalized and able to cope with all the physical, mental, and emotional demands of a busy life.

### SELF-HEALING

*The self-healing ability of the mind and body is the most powerful tool anyone can use and it can be accessed most readily during states of total relaxation. Indian head massage can help to bring about this 'light trance' state, thereby encouraging the self-healing process.*

# The way of Ayurveda

This ancient, whole-being practice, this science of life, is believed to be one of the earliest recorded systems of healing and caring for the human body, mind, and spirit.

The most important consideration in Ayurvedic medicine is a spirit and mind free from bad habits such as envy, discontent, fear, lack of creativity and purpose, and introverted self-destructive feelings of dissatisfaction. All of these can result in a body that manifests disorder and sickness. In Ayurvedic healing, as in many traditions, rather than just easing any discomfort it is most important to find the root of disharmony that results in illness and an unhappy life.

## IN TOUCH WITH THE SUBCONSCIOUS

Touch therapies are an important part of Ayurvedic medicine. They not only release tension from the body, but also place the mind and spirit in a state that withdraws from the everyday world for a while to concentrate more on the subconscious mind. The latter also governs the parasympathetic nervous system – which controls the automatic functions of the body, such as circulation and cellular renewal – keeping your body and mind going even when you are asleep. Allowing the subconscious to have its expression taps into the cellular structure of your being so that, at the most basic level, your mind and body can influence the way in which your cells repair and regenerate. In other words: this is healing at its best, most natural, and most effective.

## ENERGY FLOW

Ayurvedic practice aims to create and maintain balance between your body's digestive, elimination, and circulatory systems, calmness and creativity of mind, an open awareness of your senses, and a happy, pure, uplifted spirit. Indian head massage can assist in the smooth flow of all by stimulating energy flow in your head, face, ears, neck, and shoulders, and by promoting feelings of calm relaxation and bliss within your mind and spirit. This is a holistic therapy that works at a deep level physically, mentally, and emotionally to bring you peace, tranquillity, and calmness, and helps to open the flow of energy in your body.

## A HEALING THERAPY

Indian head massage is a part of self-help Ayurveda, which has been passed down in family traditions for many centuries. Hairdressers also use head massage as part of the hair care routine offered throughout the Middle East and now increasingly in the West. They have done much to develop head massage as a healing therapy that results in glorious, healthy hair, a calm mind, and a relaxed body.

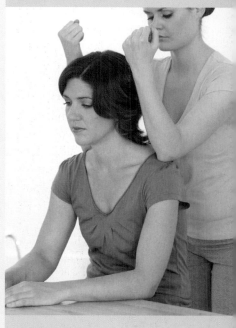

*REFLEX POINTS*
*In your head, neck, and shoulders are many reflex points and meridians which are used by other therapies to access and treat your whole being. By giving an all-over head massage you will be stimulating these areas, encouraging complete healing and harmony.*

# Meditation and visualization

For Indian head massage to succeed fully, it is important to fulfil three needs. First, your mind must be free of negative feelings and emotions such as anger or fear. Secondly, your body must free itself of disorder. Thirdly, your spirit must be at ease. Ayurvedic massage in any form aims to open up the power of the mind as well as of the body, and the use of meditation and visualization during a massage can reach far into your mental processes. Stress is reduced, enhancing creativity, focus, clarity, awareness, calmness, and connection to and understanding of others.

## DEEPENING YOUR AWARENESS

Combining Indian head massage with meditation and visualization can enable you to reach a very deep level of physical, psychological, and energetic harmony. A great deal of research has been carried out into the effects of this combination of practices, and it has been found that, once you have experienced an opening-up of spiritual and mental awareness, with regular practice you continue to grow. Intuition expands, your connection with all around you deepens, and you feel so much more in tune with the flow of life that your understanding of the role of consequences – of action and reaction – enables you to predict outcomes with such accuracy that you may feel you are experiencing an unfolding of psychic awareness. In each chapter of this book there are meditations and visualizations to help you and your partner engage the power of your minds to assist in this process.

# Mental attitude

During any massage, the mental attitudes of both you and your partner are very important. Even if you are carrying out a self-treatment, your feelings can and do affect you.

If you are angry or upset in any way, or just worrying about a problem at work or home, your massage will have an aggressive feel to it. The negativity of your energy will then be picked up by your partner, making the whole experience irritating and counterproductive. Even when you are working on yourself, if you feel anxious or that you could be better occupied elsewhere, you may find that the massage is building your worries rather than calming your mind.

## LEARN TO LET GO

If you often feel like this, it would be a good idea to practise some exercises that will allow you to enjoy being in the moment. This will enable you to drop your worries at a moment's notice, and within a few minutes refresh your mind and reduce your stress levels. In this way, you can get the best from a head massage without feeling that you are being selfish or self-indulgent. The breathing and visualization exercises on pages 36–41 can help you to balance and neutralize your mental and emotional attitudes before you start any head massage. This will enable a positive healing connection to build between you and your partner, or, if you are working alone, will calm and enrich the whole experience.

# Breathing

Breathing is one of our basic bodily functions. We take it so much for granted that it is easy to overlook the importance of correct and effective breathing.

When combined with visualization, breathing exercises can pull universal energy – *chi* – into your entire being, increasing your energy reserves and regulating and rebalancing your chakras (see right), all of which are essential for the maintenance of good health and well-being. This is why basic breathing and visualization exercises have been included throughout this book: combined with external massage, they provide a re-energizing, whole-being treatment.

As with any touch therapy, connecting with your partner is a vital part of head massage. Synchronizing your breathing and energy flows enables you to work instinctively in the areas and ways that massage is most needed, and your partner to connect with the self-healing mechanisms within their own body and mind.

## AIR QUALITY

Just as important as technique is the balance of gases in the air you breathe. Oxygen is needed for the internal combustion of food and drink, which can then be converted into energy and used in cellular renewal. The inert gases in the atmosphere – which include nitrogen, carbon dioxide, and hydrogen – are just as important, as they help to regulate the rate of the combustion as well as adding a little to the nutrients in your body.

In naturally well-balanced air you can breathe freely, without effort or much thought as to what you are

**THE CHAKRAS**
*Focused breathing can help to maintain a good balance between your chakras. These are the spinning discs of energy located throughout your body and aura. The main ones are located at the crown, 'third eye' (the point between your eyebrows), throat, heart, solar plexus, lower abdomen (hara), and the root or base. These chakras regulate the balance of our whole energy body and keep us alive.*

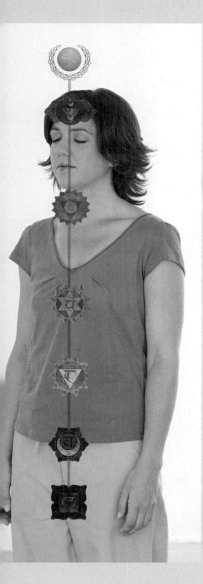

doing to your body. However, an imbalance in the ratios of the different gases caused by pollution can lead to breathing difficulties, as a result of allergic reactions to toxins in the air. In addition, you may suffer from concentration problems, headaches, tiredness, muscle fatigue, and even dizziness due to stale air containing an overload of carbon dioxide – which can also make you sleepy as it reduces the amount of oxygen your body receives.

To combat all this, it is important to spend time in a clean atmosphere and to practise breathing exercises, which will expand your lung capacity so that you can take in more of the life-giving air you need.

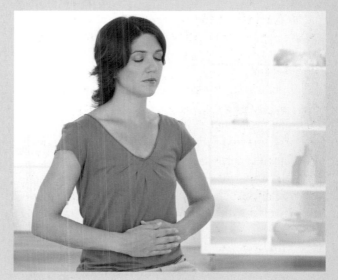

# Take care with massage

Indian head massage is very safe for use by beginners as well as those more experienced in massage. However, as with all treatments, there are some things you must look out for and treat with extra care.

- Do not use head massage in cases of injury, particularly to the neck and shoulders, as it could cause additional damage to bones, nerves, and other tissues. Even bruising should not be massaged.
- Do not massage over broken skin or any inflamed area.
- Do not massage if your partner has any infectious condition of the scalp.
- Do not use massage on those with feverish, high-temperature conditions such as colds and flu.
- Do not massage over areas containing damage to blood vessels (recognized by bruising, reddening, broken veins, localized heat, or unusual tenderness). Such damage is often age-related.
- Do not use massage on those suffering from intoxication or side-effects from drugs, as mental disturbances – such as extreme and possibly dangerous emotional release – could occur.
- Do not massage in cases of cancer.
- Take care with bone conditions such as osteoporosis.
- Take care in cases of low blood pressure, as head massage itself lowers blood pressure and this could cause fainting.
- Head massage can be very relaxing during pregnancy. However, there is a point midway along the shoulders (where you may be able to feel a tender spot) that must not be stimulated as it can produce adverse effects on blood flow to the foetus. In addition,

**MEDICAL CONDITIONS**
*Although Indian head massage can help to alleviate many clinical conditions, you should seek a physician's advice if you or your partner are suffering from any medical condition. It is not a good idea to self-diagnose, and unless a complementary therapist is medically trained they too should not attempt to diagnose a health problem. Rather, the aim of any therapy is to place the body in a state of relaxation in which repair and regeneration can occur.*

massaging on the top of the head can release emotional disturbances, so, if during pregnancy you are tearful, easily upset, angry, or in any way emotionally fragile, do not work over this area.

■ Head massage can give rise to an emotional release (see below), so in cases of mental health problems it should only be given by a professional.

## POSSIBLE AFTER-EFFECTS

In common with most complementary therapies, Indian head massage can produce after-effects. These may include aching muscles, tiredness, emotional release, and even flu-like symptoms.

When muscles have been held under tension for a long time, suddenly releasing them can result in aches and pains until they become used to working in a different way. In addition, releasing long-held toxin build-up within the muscles can give rise to muscle aches, headaches, sinus pains, and ear and eye aches.

For a short time following a massage you may feel extremely tired, emotionally as well as physically. Emotional release or upsets can be triggered easily and you may find that tears come very readily.

All of this, and other minor ailments such as colds and digestive upsets, are part of the rebalancing process and should clear up within a few days.

*HEAD MASSAGE FOR THE YOUNG, ELDERLY, OR INFIRM*
*Although Indian head massage is a very safe and gentle procedure, care needs to be taken when working on babies and children under five years old, and frail people such as the elderly, sick, or injured.*
*■ When using strokes in which pressure is exerted, use only the weight of your hands. For babies or in extremely fragile cases, use just the weight of your fingers.*
*■ Do not use hair pulling, pinching, head squeezing, or any technique that causes a degree of discomfort.*
*■ For babies, do not work over the top of the head.*
*■ Do not work over injuries, or sore or inflamed areas.*
*■ If you are using essential oils (see pages 86–89), do a skin check first as any oil (including carrier oils) can provoke an allergic reaction.*

# Using this book

In this book you will find exercises in Indian head massage, stretching, breathing, meditation, and visualization to carry you through your busy day. You can follow the basic structure and sequence of the book throughout the day, or you can choose whatever you feel will suit your mood and the circumstances of the moment.

In Chapter One you will find the basic strokes needed to give yourself and others a relaxing, rejuvenating face, head, neck, and shoulder massage in the Indian head massage tradition. There are also some breathing exercises and meditations to carry the massage through your whole being, thereby giving a holistic treatment.

There is a lot of flexibility in the way you give a head massage. If you find some of the strokes difficult or uncomfortable to use, feel free to adapt the positions of your hands or the rhythm of the stroke to suit your own and your partner's needs. Whatever *feels* good will *do* you good.

Chapter Two starts your day with some loosening stretches to warm up your muscles, and then continues with a stimulating shower massage to wake up both mind and body. Once again, there is a breathing exercise and meditation to help connect your whole being, ready for the day ahead.

Chapter Three shows you how to relieve travel discomfort and irritations with some tension-busting stretching and massage exercises. Combined with a calming breathing exercise, these will ensure you arrive at your destination ready for the challenge of the day.

The coffee-break refreshers in Chapter Four will revitalize your mind and body. These quick pick-up massage techniques and trouble-shooting headache remedies will help raise flagging spirits and provide the energy boosts you need to get you through those difficult parts of the day.

At the end of a busy day, relax and unwind in blissful solitude with a self-massage to dissolve stress and tension. Looking after yourself is a vital part of living: you cannot constantly give out, you must also replace your reserves of energy. Food and drink can only go so far in keeping you up to speed – you must also learn to release all tension build-up completely, and this takes practice, patience, and repetition. Make Chapter Five the most important part of your day.

Chapter Six provides the perfect end to the day: a full, intimate head massage to share with your partner. Here is a full sequence of massage techniques, together with meditation and breathing exercises, to connect you with your partner so that together you can give and receive a total, holistic treatment. Although it works mainly on the head, neck, and shoulders, this routine will penetrate deep within your whole being. At first, it will be important to follow the sequence as described; later, you will be able to improvise and flow with your instincts.

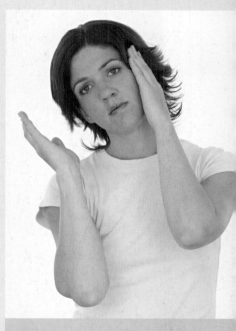

**THE FEEL-GOOD FACTOR**
*With Indian head massage, whatever feels good will do you good. Keep it smooth, flowing, effortless and, above all, relaxing.*

CHAPTER ONE

# Getting started

In Indian head massage there are a number of basic strokes that are used in many different ways. Here the strokes are described in their most common form, with some variations covered in later chapters.

There are many more ways of using these strokes, so do experiment: try to find the most pleasing ways of using touch, sequence, visualization, and energy flow to suit you and your partner.

- **Light techniques** such as holding, rocking, and stroking are used mainly to establish a very deep, energetic connection and are no less powerful than the stronger techniques. They are also the best techniques to use on babies, small children, and the elderly and/or infirm, as they have no potential to cause damage to delicate bones and tissues. However, it may not be advisable to use these strokes in cases of mental health problems, such as clinical depression, as they can release deep-held emotional issues.
- **Medium techniques** such as tapping, pushing, sliding, and rolling work mainly on the surface of the scalp, the hair, and the skin. These stimulate the flow of nutrients to the surface and help to loosen any tension within the muscles. They can also be used with stronger pressure to give a deeper, more stimulating massage.
- **Stronger techniques** such as rotations, pressure, hacking, and kneading move much more deeply into the muscles and tissues, ridding them of toxins and stimulating the circulation of blood and lymph fluids. However, if you sense any resistance to these stronger strokes, lighten their intensity and combine with lighter movements until you feel your partner relax into the massage.

# Basic strokes

The techniques described here show you the most
effective ways of positioning and working for both
giving and receiving Indian head massage.

01  02                                          03

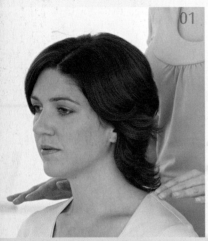
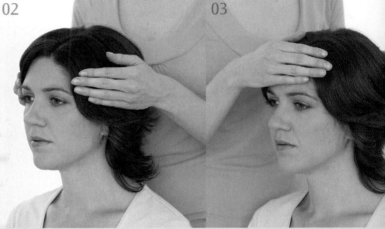

**CONNECTING**
*This is a very powerful
healing technique that
enables you to synchronize
your own energy flow with
that of your partner.*

*(01) Stand behind your
partner and focus on the
back of the head. Feel
threads of energy flowing
between you.*

*(02) Place your hands gently
on either side of the head
and synchronize your
breathing rhythm with
your partner's.*

*(03) After a few moments,
move to your partner's side
and place one hand on the
forehead and the other on
the back of the head. Again
focus for a few moments on
the energy that is flowing
between you.*

01

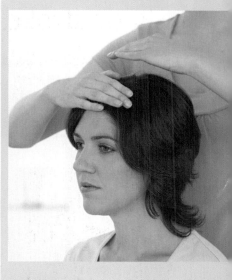

02

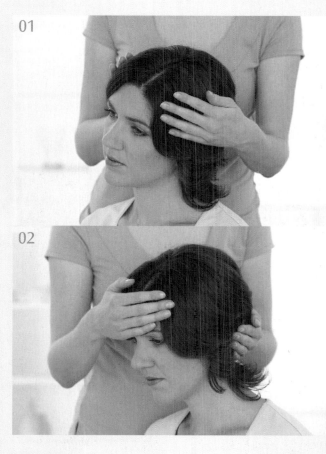

## STROKING
*This is a smooth, flowing movement that can be done with the fingers, thumbs, hands, or forearms.*

*Place your hands, fingers, thumbs, or forearms on your partner's head, neck, shoulders, or upper back and, in one smooth glide, stroke to the end position. The directions used for stroking are given in the instructions as they occur. Stroking is often repeated several times over the same area, but as a closing movement may be swept once over your partner to smooth the energy.*

## ROCKING
*This technique enables you to assess the tension in your partner's neck and shoulders before starting the treatment.*

*(01) Stand behind your partner. Place your hands on either side of the head and gently move the weight of the head from side to side.*

*(02) Move to the side of your partner. Place one hand on the forehead and the other at the base of the skull, and again gently move the head back and forth.*

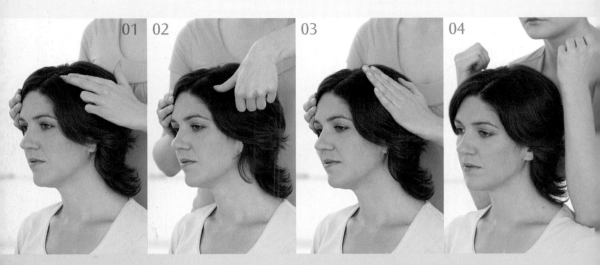

### ROTATIONS

*These circular movements can be done using your fingers, thumb, whole hand, or elbow. They help to loosen up the underlying muscles and tissues.*

*Place your fingers, thumbs, whole hand, or elbow on your partner's head, shoulders, neck, or upper back and rotate with a small circular movement.*

*(01)* **Fingers** *This movement can be done using two or more fingers. Hold your fingers about 1 cm (½ in) apart, keeping them straight.*

*Lean onto your fingers with a medium pressure and rotate them over the same spot for a few moments.*

*(02)* **Thumb** *Use one hand at a time, while holding your partner with your other hand to provide support for you both. Keeping your thumb straight and using a medium pressure, rotate your thumb for a few moments over the same spot.*

*(03)* **Hand** *This is a more gentle technique. Place your hand on your partner and, maintaining contact from the heel of your hand to the*

*fingertips, lean your body onto your hand as you rotate it over the same spot for a few moments.*

*(04)* **Elbows** *This is a very powerful technique: the sharper the angle of your elbow, the stronger the movement. Place your elbows on your partner's shoulders or upper back and rotate over the same spot for a few moments.* ***Do not use this technique on the head or the face.***

## PRESSURE

This is a still, holding technique which can be applied using your fingers, thumbs, whole hand, elbows, or forearms. The pressure used can be strong over areas such as the upper back or shoulders, and light on areas such as the face or head. Still pressure is a very useful technique that encourages the muscles to relax and let go of tension. It also assists in the smooth flow of energy throughout the body, especially if you combine it with a visualization such as the one on page 37.

(01) **Fingers** Place two or more fingers on your partner and slowly lean your body weight onto your fingers for a count of between five and ten. Release, move to the next spot, and repeat.

(02) **Thumbs** You can use one or both thumbs. Place your thumb(s) on the point of pressure and slowly lean your body weight onto it (them) for a count of between five and ten. Release, move to the next spot, and repeat.

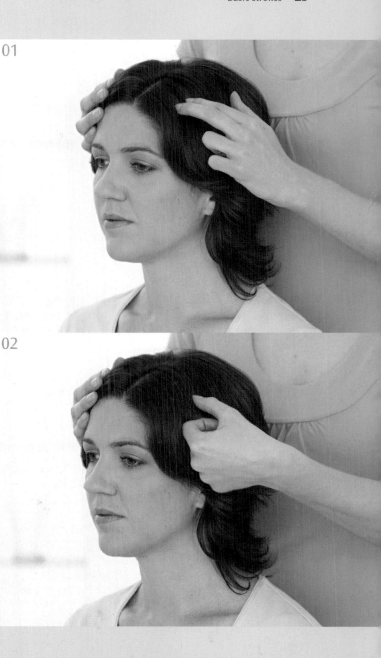

01

02

*(03)* **Hand(s)** *This is a more gentle pressure which can be used on the frail and/or elderly. You can use one or both hands. Place your hand(s) over the area and, making sure that the pressure runs right through to your fingers, lean gently and slowly onto your hand(s). Hold for a count of five and release. This can also be used as a pulsing movement in which you press and release in one smooth flow.*

*(04)* **Elbows** *This is usually used on the shoulders and upper back. Place your elbows on your partner and lean onto them for a slow count of ten. Release. The more you bend your elbows, the stronger the pressure.*

*(05)* **Forearms** *This is usually applied over the shoulders and down the upper arms. Place your forearms on your partner's shoulders and lean your weight onto them for a slow count of ten. Move down to the upper arms and press your arms inwards for a slow count of ten.*

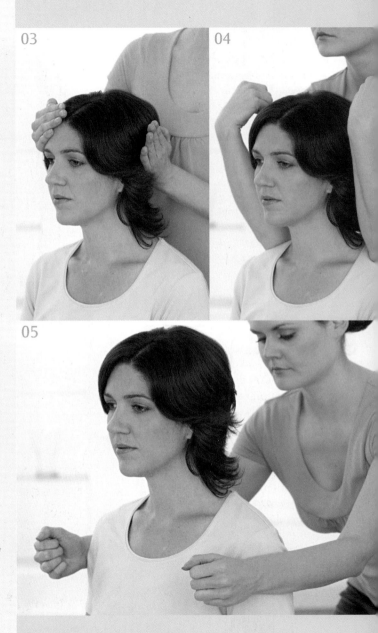

## PINCHING

*Remember: this should be a grip, not a nip. It is used to assist the movement of waste material away from the surface of the skin and back into the bloodstream, where it can then be removed by the circulatory and lymphatic systems.*

*This technique is applied by compressing flesh between your fingers and thumbs.*

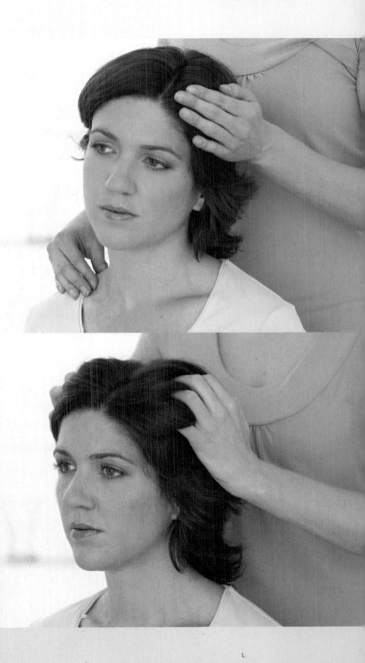

## SCRATCHING

*This technique stimulates surface circulation, helps to remove old skin and other debris from the scalp, and encourages the flow of nutrients to the hair.*

*Bend your fingers so that the tips are in line and then, in a sideways movement, lightly scratch all over your partner's head, taking care not to snag any bumps or uneven areas. You can use this technique more vigorously when both you and your partner are happy that it won't cause any damage.*

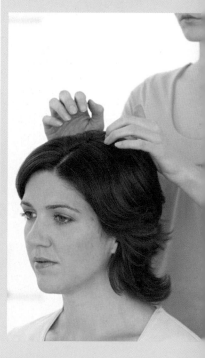

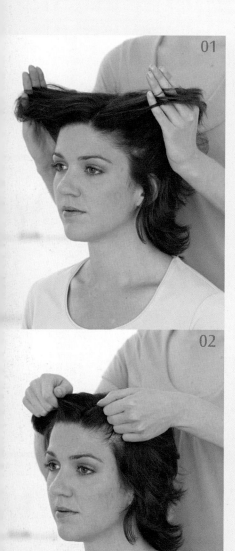

01

02

## HAIR PULLING

*This technique strengthens the hair and stimulates a good flow of nutrients to the roots. If your partner has very short hair, vigorous rotations (see page 22) will have a similar stimulating and pressure-releasing effect.*

*(01) Slide your open fingers into your partner's hair near to the roots. Close your fingers together and hold firmly while you pull your hands out to the ends of the hair. Done this way, the grip will be moderate and the action smooth.*

*(02) Another way of doing this is to take a couple of bunches of hair between the fingers and thumbs of both hands and to pull away as before. This gives a stronger grip and a harder pull, so be aware of how much feels good before pain starts. At this point, you must stop.*

## TAPPING

*This technique is excellent for energizing, as well as loosening and releasing tension. It is a percussive movement like hacking (see opposite), but is applied using the fingertips.*

*Hold your hands loosely and rapidly bounce your fingertips up and down over your partner's head, neck, and shoulders.*

## HACKING

This is a more vigorous technique than tapping, using the side of your hands with a stronger beat that works more deeply into the tissues. **Do not use on babies, children under five years old, or the elderly and/or infirm.**

Hold your hands straight and rigid. With a rapid sideways beat, moving one hand after the other, work over your partner's shoulders and upper back. This technique can also be used over the head, but the strike must be much lighter.

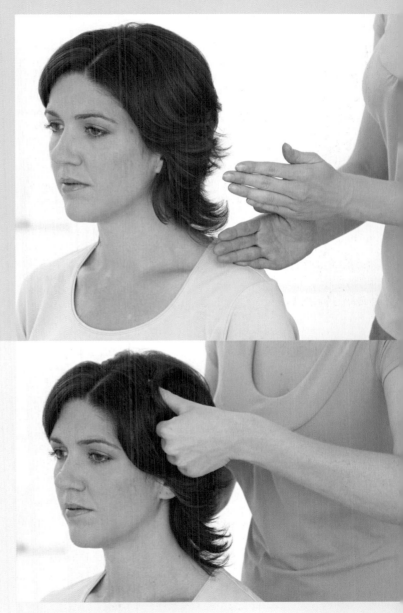

## THUMB SLIDING

This technique helps to dislodge any underlying stiffness and knotty tension in the muscles. It can be used over the whole of the head, neck, and shoulders, but not on the face as it can drag the skin.

Place your thumbs as you would for pressure (see page 23), lean onto them, and slide them in the desired direction.

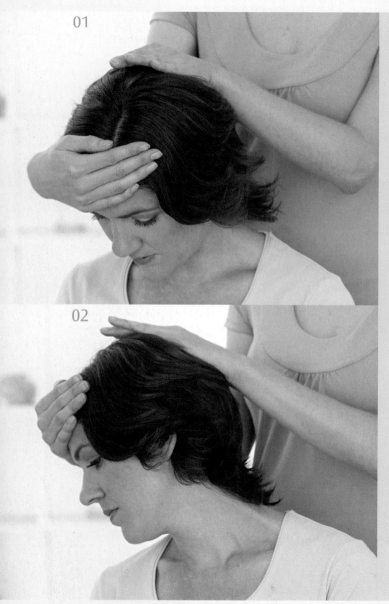

01

02

## NECK PULLING
*This is a wonderful way of loosening the muscles of the neck and shoulders, perhaps after driving or sitting for many hours at a desk or computer. Before you start, make sure your partner does not have an injury or condition that could be aggravated by the stretch.* **Do not use on babies, children under five years old, or the elderly and/or infirm.**

*(01) If your partner is seated, place one hand on the forehead and the other over the back of the head. Push the head forwards and down towards the chest.*

*(02) Very slowly stretch the head over to one side, taking it to a comfortable limit. Hold for a count of ten.*

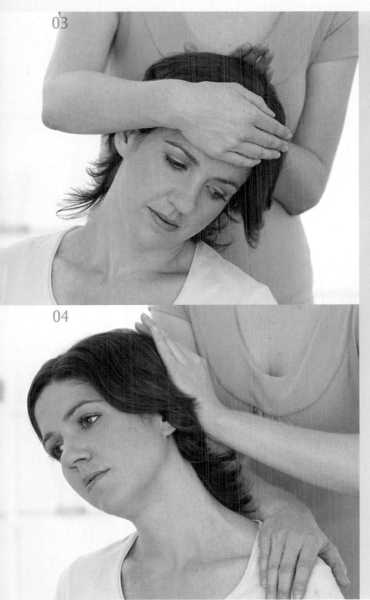

(03) *Slowly move the head back across the front and over to the other side, again taking it to a comfortable limit. You may have to adjust your hold slightly as you go. Hold for a count of ten.*

(04) *Move one hand to the shoulder and with the other stretch the head over to the side. Hold for a count of ten. Repeat on the other side. This movement must be done slowly so that you can feel if there is any resistance.*
  *If your partner's neck is particularly stiff, take the stretch to a comfortable level and then gently rock the head to encourage further release of any tense muscles and an increase in the stretch. After a few more treatments, you will probably find that the neck will relax and loosen.*

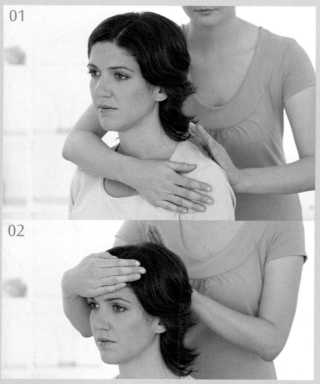

### SQUEEZING
*This technique is similar to pinching (see page 25), but it covers a larger area and the grip can be stronger as there is no chance of nipping a nerve. It is very good for removing toxins from the skin and underlying flesh.*

*Place your hands over the area to be squeezed (usually the shoulders or upper arms). Grasp the flesh firmly in your hands by squeezing your fingers towards the heels of your hands.*

### PUSHING
*This stroke is usually applied with the heel of the hand, but in small areas it can be done with the fingers. It is a deep, releasing movement which works right down to the roots of tension in muscle tissue. Pushing is very good for releasing toxins from muscles and other tissue.*

*(01) Using the resistance of your partner's body, lean your weight onto one hand and then slide it slowly across the shoulders.*

*(02) If you are working on the head, use one hand to brace the head while you push with the other.*

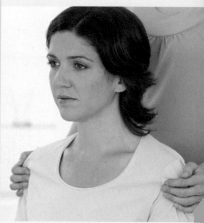

01

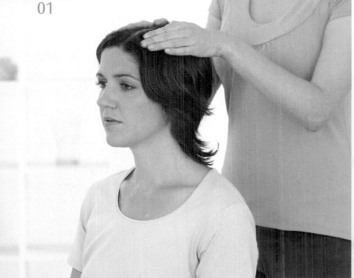

02

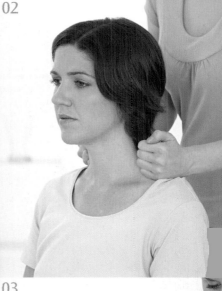

03

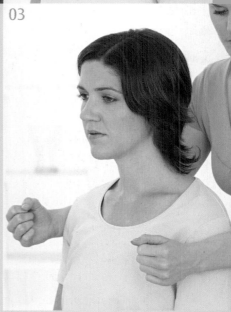

### SLIDING

This movement will aid circulation and muscle release. It is also very useful for linking one technique to the next, to create a smooth, flowing treatment. The stroke can be applied with the palms of the hands, fists, or forearms.

Run your hands (fists, or forearms) over the area, keeping up a constant moderate pressure.

(01) **Hands** Place your hands on your partner and slide them over the area that is to be worked.

(02) **Fists** Place your closed fists on your partner and, using strong pressure, slide them over the area that is to be worked.

(03) **Forearms** Place your forearms on your partner and slide them over the area to be worked. If you do this with open hands, the pressure is moderate. Closing your fists enables you to increase the pressure.

### ROLLING

*With this technique you can cover a large area quickly to relax and release tension. For those new to massage, it is excellent for building confidence in bodywork.*

*Apply firm pressure with the heels of your hands and roll the pressure along your hand to the fingertips. Repeat as necessary.*

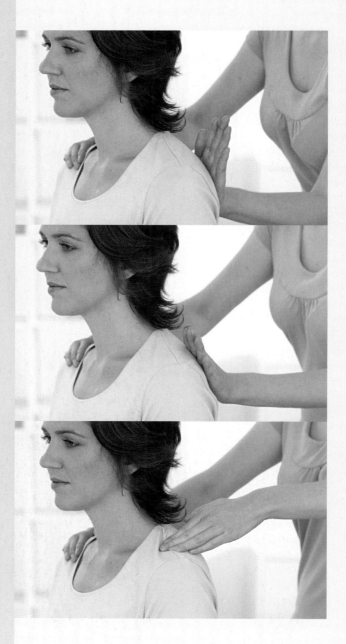

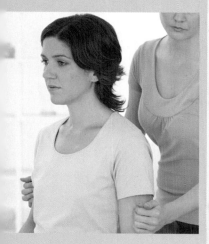

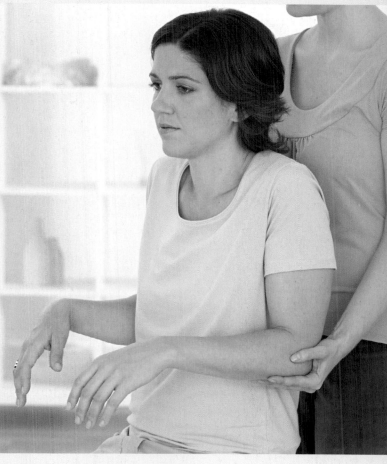

## SQUEEZING AND PULLING

This is a deep, invigorating movement which releases toxin build-up from muscle fibres. You can apply it with one hand or both.

With one hand, squeeze as in the squeezing technique (see page 30) and slowly pull the flesh away in a sideways direction. At the end of the pull, allow the flesh to slide from your grasp under tension. If you are using two hands, interlock your fingers and place the heels of your hands on either side of, say, the shoulder (see page 120). Grasp the flesh firmly, then pull upwards and release, as before.

## SHOULDER LIFT AND RELEASE

This technique quickly relaxes the whole of your partner's upper back and shoulders. **Do not use on babies, children under five years old, or the elderly and/or infirm.**

Stand behind your partner and put both your hands under the elbows. Take a firm hold and lift straight up, then quickly release your grip, allowing the shoulders to drop.

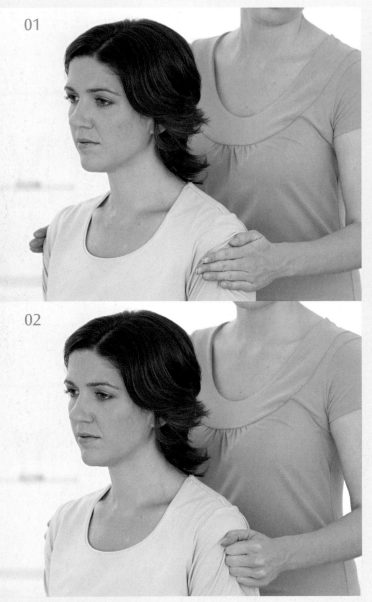

### FRICTION

This is a brisk rubbing motion which can be done with an open hand or fist. It is very useful for warming up muscles, as well as for releasing tension.

(01) **Open hand** Support your partner with one hand, then place your open hand over the area to be worked and, with either a circular motion or a back-and-forth movement, rub briskly.

(02) **Fist** Support your partner with one hand. Hold your other hand in a fist and, with either a circular motion or a back-and-forth movement, rub briskly.

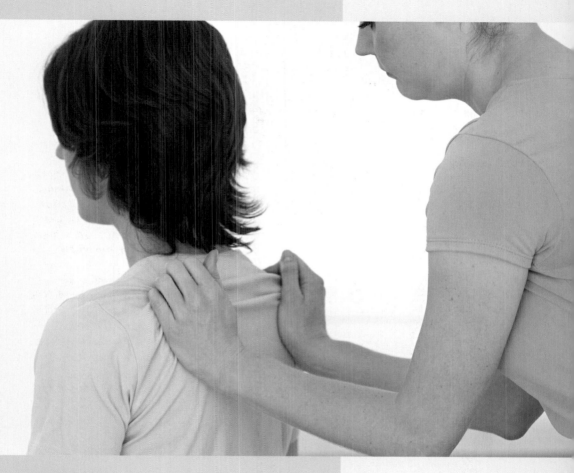

## KNEADING
This is a very deep and relaxing technique which loosens long-held tension in large muscles. It should be used over the upper back, arms, and shoulders.

Make this repetitive action by pushing the heels of your hands quickly towards your fingers, in a similar way to kneading dough. This movement massages the tissues strongly and deeply.

# Breathing exercises

Daily breathing exercises will help to keep your body, mind, and spirit well tuned and in good health. They will increase your lung capacity, enhance physical stamina, improve the condition of your skin, hair, and nails, increase energy levels, improve concentration, and stimulate mental processes. Focused breathing can also reduce levels of pain when needed and help to rid your body of toxins.

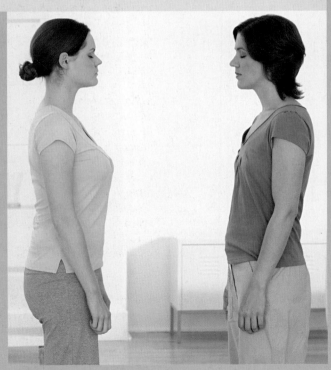

**CIRCULAR BREATHING**
*This breathing exercise balances the main chakras of your body. It can be used to synchronize your breathing with that of your partner, which will also 'tune in' your energies to each other. The openings of the chakras are down the front of your body and the roots are at the back. While inhaling, you will visualize your breath moving down the front of your body, and while exhaling you will visualize it moving up the back of your body.*

*If you are working with a partner, stand either behind or facing them as you synchronize your breathing and energies. Throughout, breathe in through your nose and out through your mouth.*

*Close your eyes and imagine a softly glowing light coming down from the universe to your transpersonal point – situated about 1 m (3 ft) above your head. Place the tip of your tongue just behind your front teeth. This will complete the power cycle which you are about to energize.*

*Breathe in – fill this point with light.*

*Breathe out – move the light down to your crown chakra.*

*Breathe in – feel a clear white light filling this chakra.*

*Breathe out – move the light down to your 'third eye' chakra.*

*Breathe in – feel this chakra glowing with an indigo light.*

*Breathe out – move the light down to your throat chakra.*

*Breathe in – feel a soft blue light filling this chakra.*

*Breathe out – move the light down to your heart chakra. At this point you may sense a softly glowing turquoise light midway between your throat and heart chakras. If so, take another breath here to acknowledge its presence, then move on.*

*Breathe in – feel a gentle green light filling your heart chakra.*

*Breathe out – move the light downwards to your solar plexus.*

*Breathe in – feel an energizing yellow light filling this chakra.*

*Breathe out – move the light down to your* hara *(lower abdomen).*

*Breathe in – feel this chakra filling with an orange light that grounds your energy within the powerhouse of your chakra system.*

*Breathe out – move the light down to your root chakra.*

*Breathe in – feel this chakra filling with a deep, fiery red light. Take a couple of breaths to build this fire. See its volcanic power. The cycle now begins.*

*Breathe in – gather the power within this chakra.*

*Breathe out – move the power up your spine to the crown chakra in one smooth sweep.*

*Breathe in – draw the power down the front of your chakras to your root chakra.*

*Breathe out – again move the power up your spine to your crown chakra.*

*Repeat this cycle for about 15 breaths. Open your eyes and move into the massage.*

**WATERFALL BREATHING**
*This exercise clears and purifies your energy system, helping to ground your emotions and remove any negative thoughts and feelings which could intrude on the connection between you and your partner. If you are doing a self-treatment, this exercise would also be very helpful in neutralizing any negativity that has clung to you during the day. You can use it any time you feel stressed, angry, fearful, tired, or in any way negative. It will boost your energy levels and refresh your mind.*

*Imagine you are standing under a silvery waterfall.*

*Breathe in and feel the water washing over and through you.*

*Breathe out and feel all your tension, tiredness, and negative feelings washing away, down into the earth.*

*Continue this cycle of breathing until you feel clear and freshened.*

## CONNECTING AND CHANNELLING HEALING WITH A PARTNER

*Connecting with your partner is a vital part of any healing massage. To do this, first of all you and your partner need to be in stillness together.*

*Place your hands on your partner and breathe slowly and evenly as you visualize a bright, healing light surrounding you both. This light can be white, pink, soft yellow, blue, or violet. Don't worry about directing the light at this stage – just enjoy its calming and healing properties. Then move into one of the breathing exercises described on pages 36–37.*

*The breathing exercise will help you to meld the healing energies of the universe with you and your partner. Then, to channel these energies, you will need to be open and objective. See yourself as a conduit through which the healing light flows from the universe, down through the top of your head into your hara (lower abdomen), then back up around your shoulders, and out through your hands into your partner.*

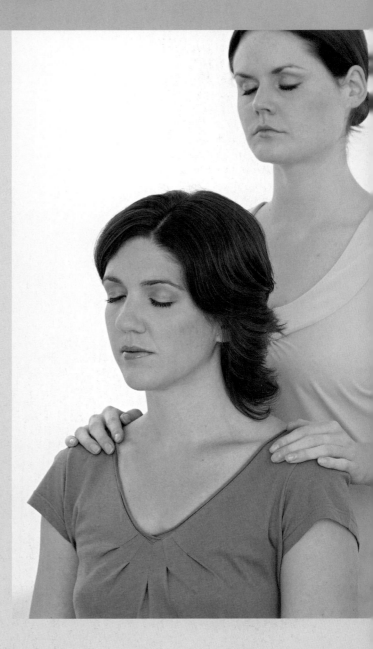

## CONNECTING WITH YOUR INNER SELF AND YOUR PARTNER – CENTRING

To get the very best out of any head massage, be it a self-treatment or with a partner, you will need to centre yourself and make the connection with universal energies before commencing. You will then be tapping into the most powerful of healing processes.

Here is a simple way to make that connection. Throughout, breathe in through your nose and out through your mouth. Breathe slowly and deeply – for a count of six on the in-breath and eight on the out-breath – for a few moments. At the same time, imagine yourself on a great wheel of energy coming down from the universe, through your (and your partner's) body, into the earth, and then flowing back up into the sky.

**For yourself** Sit quietly with your hands over your hara (lower abdomen).

Breathe in – pull the energy down and through your body to your hara.

Breathe out – push the energy out through your feet,

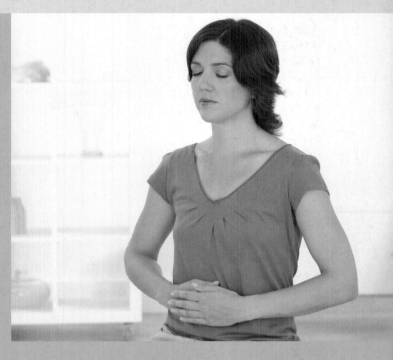

deep into the earth, and back up into the sky.

Continue this cycle for eight to ten breaths and really feel yourself part of this universal wheel. Try to hold on to that feeling of connection while you are working with the massage.

**With a partner** Stand behind your partner and place your hands on the shoulders.

Breathe in – pull the energy down through your body to your hara.

Breathe out – pull the energy up through your body, out into your hands, and into your partner. Then continue visualizing this flow moving down through your partner, into the earth, and back up into the sky, to form a great wheel of energy.

Continue with this cycle for eight to ten breaths, feeling your and your partner's energies as one, and at one with the universe.

### VISUALIZATION AND INTENTION

As well as rebalancing your emotions, visualization techniques can help to focus and direct your healing energies. Any massage can be more deeply effective if you combine the physical moves with a focused visualization of the effect the massage is having on the tissues beneath the surface. For example, imagine muscles loosening and relaxing or toxins easing their way out of the body – this really does work. Many times I have had the person I've been working on tell me that they felt a deep shift of long-held stiffness or pain suddenly sliding away, even when my touch has been very light.

A very important part of healing is your intention while you are working. Basically, intention is a conscious combination of a positive mental attitude and visualization, carried through with a loving, caring focus. Even if you are working on yourself, you should be careful to use well-directed intention. Your energy system is like any other muscle: you intend your hand to move and it moves – you don't have to make an effort to do this, you just do it. It is the same with the intention you put behind your massage: it works best if you don't try too hard. Just do it. Intend good health and well-being for your partner and it will be there. It is as simple as that. If you intend the hair to be glossy and supple, or the shoulders to be relaxed and strong, visualize just that and the healing energy and your massage will follow, giving the kind of treatment that will produce exactly that result.

***Example*** *Your partner has a stuffy headache.*

*Stand behind your partner and make the connection (see page 38), this time with your hands on the head.*

*Imagine a healing white light coming down from the stars, through the top of your head, and through your body to your* hara *(lower abdomen). Pull the light back up your body and into your hands. Feel them glowing in the light.*

*Imagine this light flowing from your hands into your partner's head, into the hair, through the roots, into the scalp, and into the brain. Imagine the light filling the brain, face, ears, and neck.*

*See the light glowing brighter and brighter, until your hands are filled with this brightly glowing ball of light.*

*Imagine the headache as a grey area within the light. See the light working on the grey area, transforming it into light.*

*Feel your hands draining away any existing pain within the light.*

*This will work on any area of the body, even if your hands are only placed on the head or shoulders. Just direct the light towards the disturbed area.*

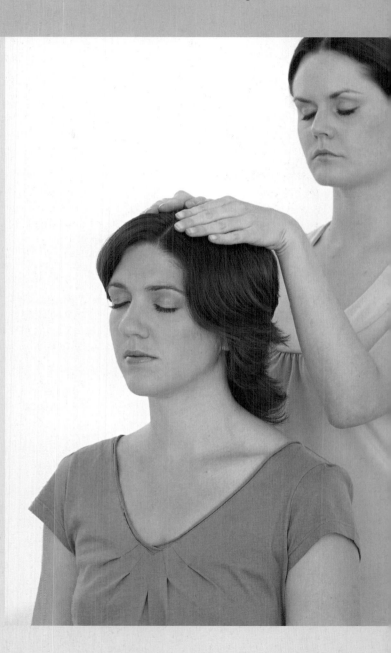

# CHAPTER TWO

# Preparing for the day

Although you may feel warm and cosy in your bed, after hours of stillness and relaxation your muscles need to be awakened gently. This 'waking up' of your muscles also helps to wake up your mind.

A few minutes spent doing stretches and breathing exercises will loosen your body and increase mental clarity. If you combine breathing with visualization, you will find that your energy levels increase and your mind becomes more agile and creative.

Head massage in the shower helps to clear and loosen debris, dirt, and flaking skin, releases stiffness in your neck, and improves the condition of your hair. However, you need to take care, as wet hair is more easily damaged than dry hair, so the massage (particularly near the roots) should be lighter and gentler than if you were massaging over dry hair. Try to use the more vigorous techniques before you step into the shower.

The final sweeping movement (see page 52) will help to rebalance your surface energy. Many energy workers and healers use this movement, together with the burning of purifying herbs or oils and visualization, as part of their dawn preparations to cleanse, equalize, and stabilize the surface energy of the body and aura ready for the day. If you wish to combine the sweeping with purifying herbs, incense, or oils, stand in the vapour of burning sage (not to be used during pregnancy) or frankincense and waft it over your body and aura with the sweeping sequence.

# Wake-up stretches

These stretches are more beneficial the more slowly they are performed. This not only eases the muscles out of sleep in a way that will not jerk or overreach them, but also concentrates maximum effort and awareness into the movement. At all times, breathe slowly, deeply, and evenly. This deep breathing will help to lower your blood pressure and sharpen your mind. Good oxygenation of the sight and sound receptors in the brain can also help to sharpen eyesight and hearing.

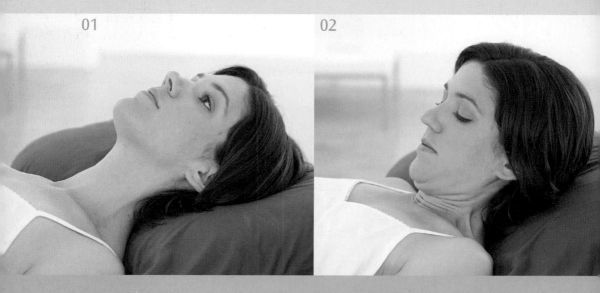

01

02

(01) Before you even get out of bed, start by stretching your head up along the pillow as far as you can reach. Feel your neck lengthening and the scalp at the back of your head releasing. Hold the stretch for a count of ten. Relax.

(02) Very slowly, lift your head from the pillow and move your chin down towards your chest. Hold for a count of ten. Relax.

*(03) Slowly roll your head over to the left until your face touches the pillow. Hold for a count of ten, then relax. Return your head to the centre with your chin on your chest and continue the roll over to the right side. Hold for a count of ten, then relax.*

*(04) In a slow rotation, move your arms out to the side and up over your head, extending your fingers as far as they will go. As you move your arms up over your head, clench and release your hands several times. Each time, explore the feeling in the muscles from your shoulders to your fingertips as you stretch outwards. Slowly return your arms to your sides. Relax.*

*(05) With your arms by your sides, press your palms into the bed and, using your hands as support, arch your back upwards as far as you can go. Hold for a count of ten. Relax.*

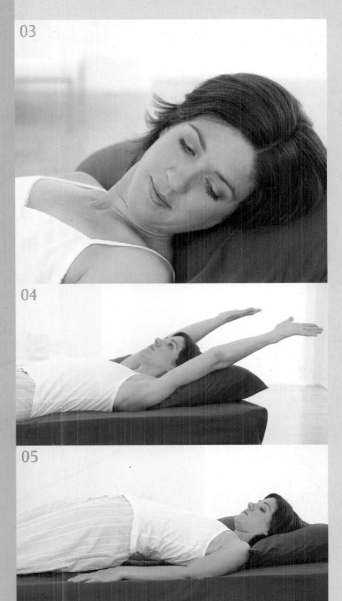

03

04

05

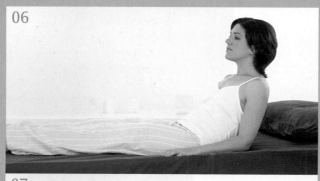

(06) Slowly, moving from the buttocks, lift your upper body to a sitting position, keeping your back as straight as possible as you go. The slower you can do this, the better.

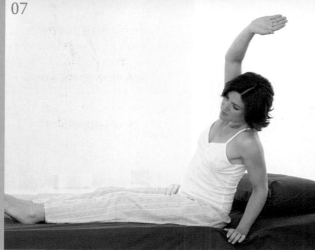

(07) Raise one arm above your head and, keeping your back straight, bend your body over to the opposite side, stretching your raised arm as far as you can. When you have reached your limit, hold the position for a count of ten. Slowly return to the upright sitting position and relax. Repeat to the other side, and relax.

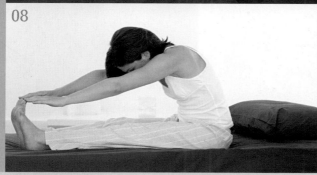

(08) Bring your arms to the front, hands parallel to your legs. Slowly drop forwards, stretching down towards your toes. Try to relax into this stretch, allowing your body weight to extend the stretch to your toes. Hold for a count of ten. Relax.

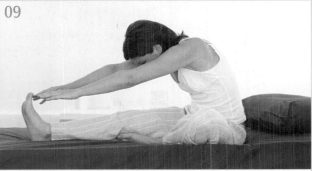

(09) Sit upright and bend one leg so that your foot touches the knee of the opposite leg and your other knee is lowered as close to the bed as possible. Raise your arms and slowly drop forwards to touch the toes of your extended leg. Hold for a count of ten. Relax. Repeat with the other leg bent, then relax.

(10) Sit upright and rotate your feet ten times clockwise and ten times anticlockwise. Finish by wriggling your toes.

Now move straight into the squeezing sequence on page 48.

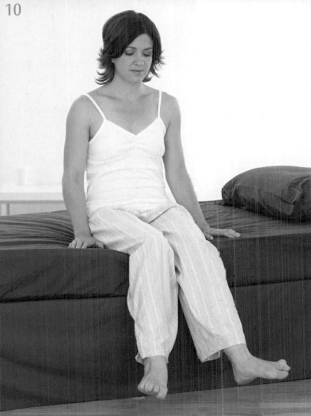

# Wake-up massages

This massage sequence continues the steady reawakening. After hours of relative stillness, stagnation builds up within your brain and body. This massage routine will help to get you up to speed quickly and effectively.

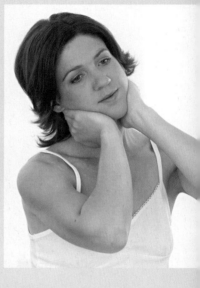

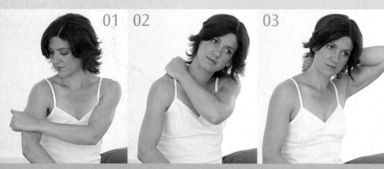

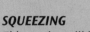

**SQUEEZING**
*This routine will help you to release any waste matter or toxins that have built up in the muscles of your arms, shoulders, and neck.*

*(01) Start by squeezing the flesh on the outer side of one forearm by working the fingers of your other hand against the heel of that hand, grasping firmly and pull away. Move your hand to just above the elbow, then repeat the squeeze and pull*

*away. Move your hand a hand's width higher, then repeat the squeeze and pull. Move and repeat until you have reached your shoulder.*

*(02) Work along your shoulder in the same way, then up into the fleshy area on the side of your neck. Repeat the sequence on your other arm, shoulder, and neck.*

*(03) Finally, grasp the flesh at the back of your neck and pull away.*

**ROCKING**
*This simple movement will free up any stiffness held in your neck muscles. It is also a good technique to use at any time of day if you have been sitting in cramped conditions for any length of time.*

*Place your hands on either side of your jaw and rock your head from side to side for a few moments, to loosen up the whole of your neck.*

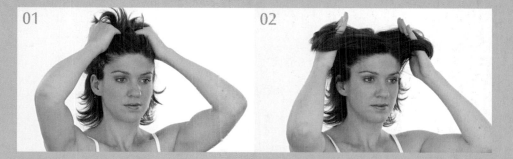

### HAIR PULLING

This strong technique increases the flow of nutrients to your hair roots, scalp, nerves – even your brain. If you have very short hair, see page 26 for an alternative suggestion.

(01) Slide both hands from your forehead into your hair, close to the roots. Take hold of your hair and shake back and forth for a few moments. Repeat all over your head.

(02) Slide your fingers into your hair, close them together, hold tightly, and slide your fingers out towards the ends of the hair. Repeat all over your head. Relax.

### BREATHING BRIGHT LIGHT

This exercise is very invigorating. It rapidly increases the levels of oxygen within your body and brain, helping to flush out toxins and waste matter and revitalizing every cell. It is the spark plug of your day.

Stand on the floor, well balanced with your feet apart and knees slightly bent. Throughout, breathe in through your nose and out through your mouth.

Breathe in – imagine you are standing within a pillar of bright light.

Breathe out – imagine your mind and body spreading outwards until you feel about 3 m (10 ft) wide.

Breathe in – feel the light filling your body.

Breathe out – feel the light within you growing brighter.

Continue this cycle of breathing – filling your body with light on the in-breath and building the brightness of the light on the out-breath – for about 20 breaths. Relax.

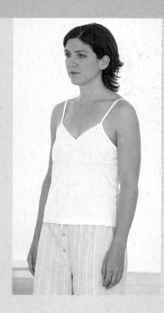

# Showering

When you are taking a shower, imagine the water flowing freely through you as well as over you, moving all the night's sleepiness out and away. Flowing water earths static energy and clears your channels. Feel it brightening your whole being, opening you to the creativity that is all around.

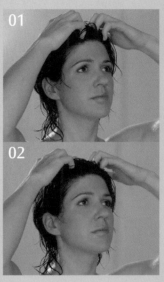

01

02

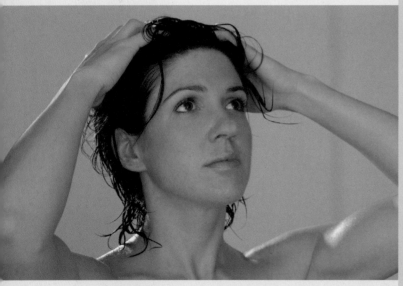

### SCRATCHING

*This technique helps to release any dead cells on your scalp and stimulate the flow of nutrients to the surface of your skin.*

*(01) Hold your fingers loosely bent and in a line. Starting on the centre of your head, at the hairline, scratch lightly back and forth with your nails, taking care not to snag your scalp.*

### SHAMPOOING

*While working the shampoo through your hair, take the opportunity to massage your scalp with firm, rotating movements of your fingers.*

*Cover your whole head and neck in this way. Remember that wet hair is damaged more easily than dry hair, so the massage here should be light and free flowing.*

*(02) Move your hands to about 2 cm (¾ in) apart and repeat the scratching. Repeat until you have covered your whole head.*

## KNUCKLE RUB

*These powerful movements work to release deeply held tension and stress.*

*(01) Hold your hand in a firm fist. Starting on the hand of your other arm, rub strongly all over with your knuckles. Move up your arm, rubbing strongly. Repeat for the other hand and arm.*

*(02) Rub all over your shoulders and neck with a strong, brisk action.*

*(03) When you reach your head, you can use both fists together. Rub briskly, with light pressure.*

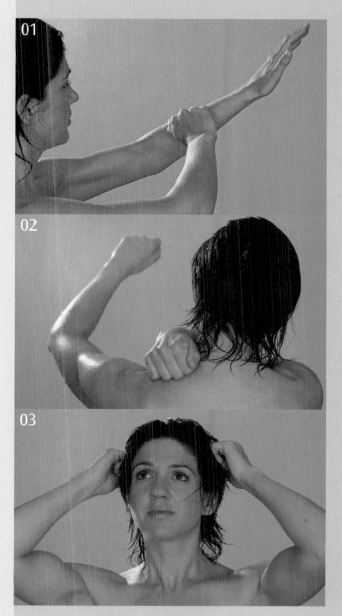

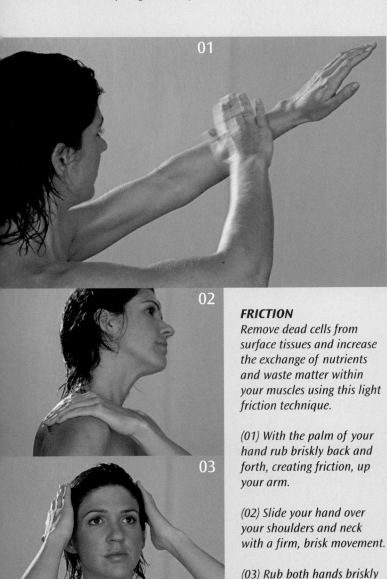

**01**

**02**

**03**

## SWEEPING
*This technique can be carried out dry as well as under a shower.*

*(01) Starting with both hands on the top of your head, lightly and quickly sweep them down either side.*

*(02) Next, sweep the back of your head.*

*(03) Sweep your hands gently over your face.*

*(04) Place your right hand on the back of your neck and sweep it down your left arm from neck to fingertips. Repeat the sweep with your left hand over your right arm.*

*(05) Move to your throat and chest area and sweep your hands down the front of your body, right to your feet.*

*(06) Move to your back and, using the backs of your hands (as you may find you can reach higher up your back this way), sweep quickly down your back to your feet.*

## FRICTION
*Remove dead cells from surface tissues and increase the exchange of nutrients and waste matter within your muscles using this light friction technique.*

*(01) With the palm of your hand rub briskly back and forth, creating friction, up your arm.*

*(02) Slide your hand over your shoulders and neck with a firm, brisk movement.*

*(03) Rub both hands briskly over your head together with light pressure. Repeat the sequence on the other side.*

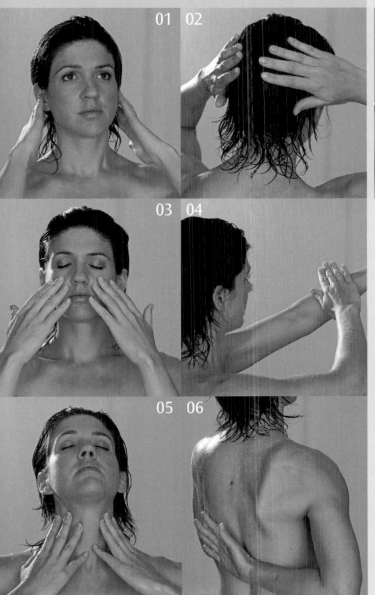

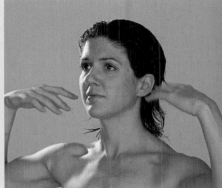

### SHAKING

This final exercise is quite enlivening and will set you up for the day ahead.

Climb out of the shower and, before you dry off, shake your hands. Carry this shaking up your arms and through your entire body and head, continuing for a few moments until you feel nicely invigorated.

# CHAPTER THREE

# On the move

**Whether it be daily commuting or long-haul journeys, travelling involves time spent in often cramped conditions with stale air, tiring traffic situations, and sometimes annoying co-travellers!**

**H**ead massage can relieve much of the discomfort, increase your alertness, restore calm patience and concentration, and help to ensure that you have a safer and more pleasant trip.

During a long journey you may become very stiff and tired. On trains or planes, take a walk to a quiet area and loosen up. If you are driving, park the car and take a short stroll, breathing deeply with long, cool breaths to release your tension. The routines in this chapter will help to free up tight muscles, relax your back, shoulders, neck and scalp, and relieve tired eyes. They may take only a few minutes, but will release any stiffness in your body, refresh your mind, and calm your emotions.

The simple breathing exercise will help to release tension in stressful situations, such as busy traffic or where buses or trains are running late. It will also serve to re-oxygenate your brain, helping you to stay alert and free from traffic panic. You should become familiar with the technique before you attempt it while driving, as otherwise it could distract your attention.

### CALMING BREATH

This calming breathing and visualization exercise relieves nervous tension and clears your thoughts. It is very useful in any tense situations you may find yourself in during the day, including when dealing with difficult relationships. Just surround yourself with the bubble and visualize the problem or person outside its walls, so that you can view everything calmly, objectively, and creatively. Imagine all of your tension draining away through the walls of the bubble, which will then keep it away from you. You will no longer be stressed by any external irritations. Enjoy your day.

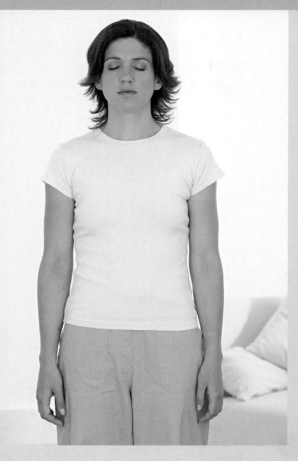

Imagine a large bubble surrounding you. You are going to fill this bubble with a soft, calming glow that will enable you to disconnect from any irritating situations you may encounter during your travels. Throughout, breathe in through your nose and out through your mouth.

Breathe in – draw a soft blue light into your hara (lower abdomen). Feel your abdomen filling with this light.

Breathe out – push this light out upwards and sideways to fill your body, your mind, and the bubble.

Continue this cycle of breathing, slowly filling your body, your mind, and the bubble with soft, calming blue light.

On the in-breath, deepen the intensity of the light.

On the out-breath, see all your tension being drawn out to the very edges of the bubble and feel it slipping out through the walls.

# Neck and shoulder workout

The following two routines will bring instant relief to
tense neck and shoulder muscles, plus a host of other
benefits, including relaxing your scalp, and easing
pressure headaches and eyestrain.

01

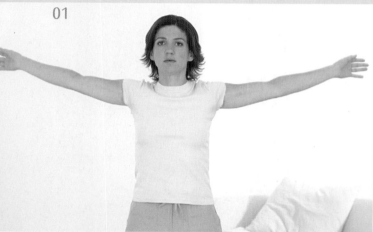

02

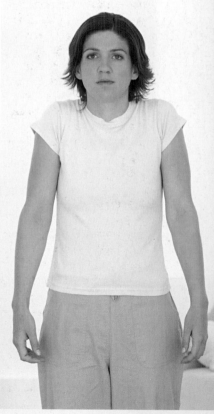

### SHOULDER AND NECK RELEASE

*This exercise loosens tension
in your shoulders, neck, and
back. It also eases stiffness
in the joints, re-oxygenates
the mind and body, clears
stuffy headaches, stretches
muscles, and frees up your
whole body.*

*(01) Swing your arms in wide
circles at either side.*

*(02) To release your back and
shoulder muscles, hunch up
your shoulders towards your
ears and release quickly four
to five times.*

03

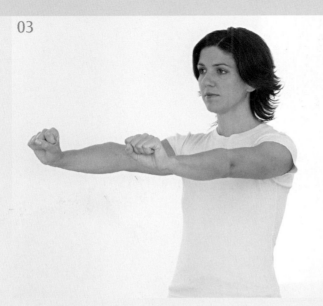

04

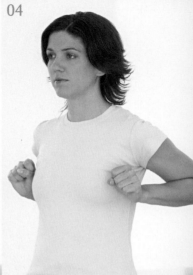

05

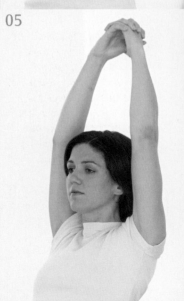

*(03) Breathe in – push your clenched fists straight out in front of you.*

*(04) Breathe out – pull back and push your elbows backwards as far as you can. Do this fairly rapidly four to five times.*

*(05) Clasp your hands together in front of your body. Straighten your arms and raise them above your head. Take your arms back as far as you can manage comfortably. Hold for a slow count of ten and relax. Repeat three times.*

06

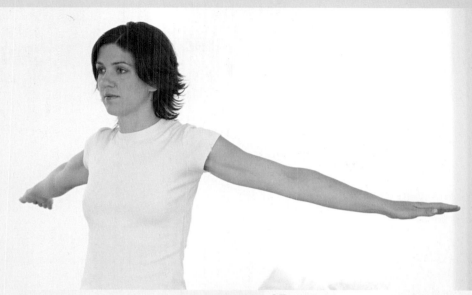

(06) Hold your hands out in front of you, palms down. With a slow swimming action, move your hands out to the sides and back as far as you can. Hold for a slow count of ten. Return your arms to the front. Repeat three times.

(07) Clasp your hands behind your back. Straighten your arms and, keeping your back straight, raise them behind you as far as you can manage comfortably. Hold for a slow count of ten and relax. Repeat three times.

07

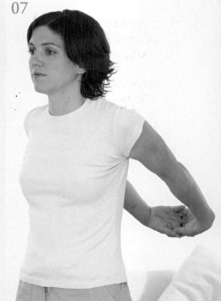

01  02 03

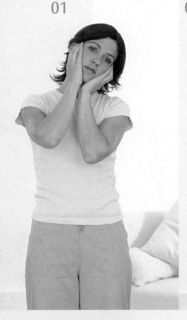 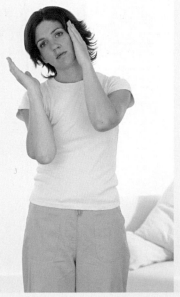 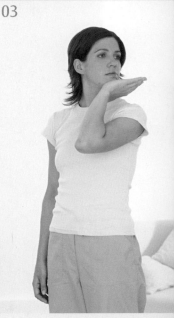

### NECK RELEASE
*These stretches relieve tension in your neck and help to reduce eyestrain and facial aches. The squeezing will help to refresh muscles and increase blood and nutrient circulation, particularly to your brain.*

*(01) Hold your head with both hands and slowly drop it to the left until it reaches your shoulder. Hold this position*

*for a count of ten. Take your head down and across your chest to the other side. Hold again for a count of ten.*

*(02) Bring your head back to the centre and lightly toss it from hand to hand. If your neck is really relaxed this should be a light movement.* **Do not toss your head if you feel any resistance or sharp, painful discomfort.**

*(03) If your neck is very stiff and you find it painful or uncomfortable to toss the head from hand to hand, instead you can loosen up your neck by pushing your chin as far as you can, first to one side then to the other, with your hand. This will allow you to feel the limits of your neck's flexibility and, with practice, will increase its stretch and flexibility.*

04        05        06        07

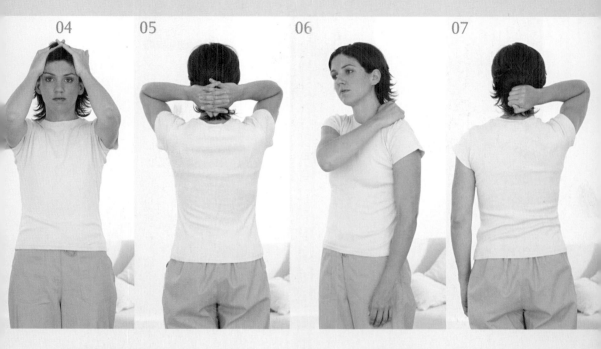

(04) Place your hands on either side of your head, level with your temples. Interlock your fingers and squeeze the heels of your hands together, keeping the tension in an upwards direction. The pressure should be quite strong. Hold the squeeze for about ten seconds, then, keeping the pressure constant, slide your hands upwards so that they meet above your head. Move your hands back about a palm's width and repeat.

(05) Keep repeating the squeeze, moving your hands backwards until you reach the base of your neck.

(06) Using one hand on the opposite shoulder, squeeze your fingers against the heel of your hand. Move a palm's width along your shoulder and repeat. Repeat for the other shoulder. **Do not use this technique during pregnancy (see page 14).**

(07) Place one hand on the back of your neck and squeeze the fingers towards the heel of your hand. Pull back, allowing the flesh to slide through your hand.

# Face, head, and neck workout

This routine loosens and freshens up your facial muscles and relaxes your jaw, which will help to reduce nervous tension and irritability. *Do not use strong pressure on any injury or site of surgery, such as sinus drainage implants.*

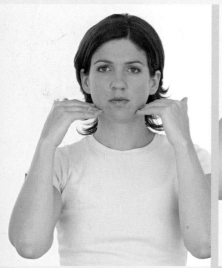

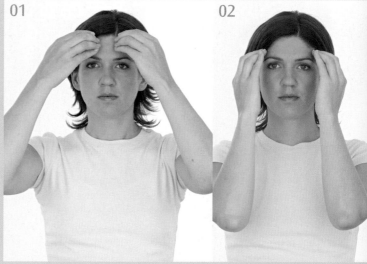

**FLICKING THE SKIN**
*This light, sharp, rapid movement stimulates blood flow to the skin's surface.*

*With your hands either side of your face, work upwards all over your face flicking the skin with your fingertips with loose movements.*

**TAPPING**
*Softer and more gentle than flicking, this technique works more deeply into the muscle tissue to stimulate and tone.*

*(01) Hold your fingertips in a vertical line at the centre of your forehead. Tap outwards until you reach the temples. Repeat three to four times.*

*(02) Place your fingers along the top of your eyebrows. Tap over the brows and outwards towards the temples. Repeat three to four times.*

03  04

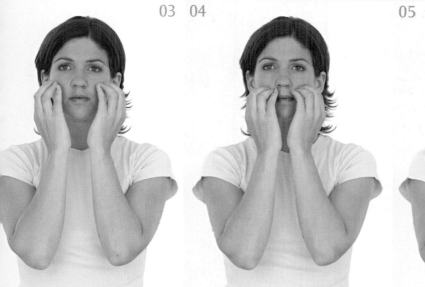

05

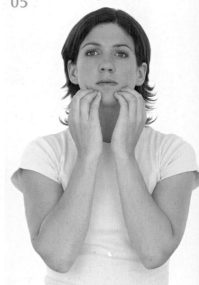

(03) Place your fingers in a horizontal line along your cheekbones. Tap along the bones towards your ears. Repeat three to four times.

(04) Place your fingers in a horizontal line under your nose. Tap across your upper jawline towards your ears. Repeat three to four times.

(05) Place your fingers under your mouth, with little fingers touching. Tap along your lower jawline towards your ears. Repeat three to four times.

(06) Place your fingers in a horizontal line at the back of your neck, fingertips touching. Tap around to the front of your neck. Repeat three to four times.

06

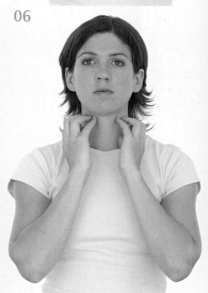

01 02 03

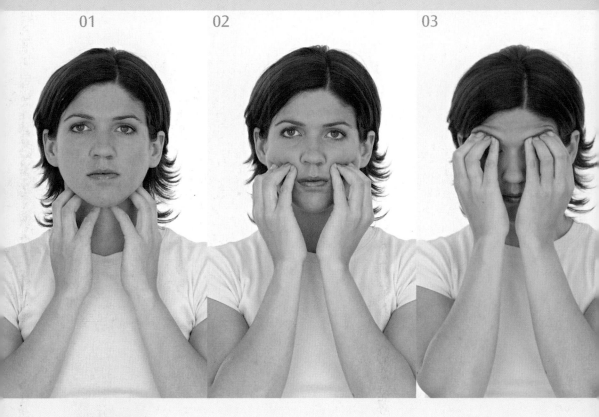

### PRESSURE

*This technique stimulates areas of the face that will help to release whole mind/body tensions, relieve tired eyes, release your jaw, and reduce sinus problems and frontal headaches.*

*(01) Place your fingertips just under your lower jawline. Drop the weight of your head onto your fingers and press in an upwards direction. Hold for a count of ten.*

*(02) Place your fingertips along the line of your upper jawline. Drop your head forwards onto your fingers and press the fingers in an upwards direction. Hold for a count of ten.*

*(03) Place your fingertips along the line of your eyebrows. Drop the weight of your head forwards onto your fingers and press in an upwards direction. Hold for a count of ten.*

04    05

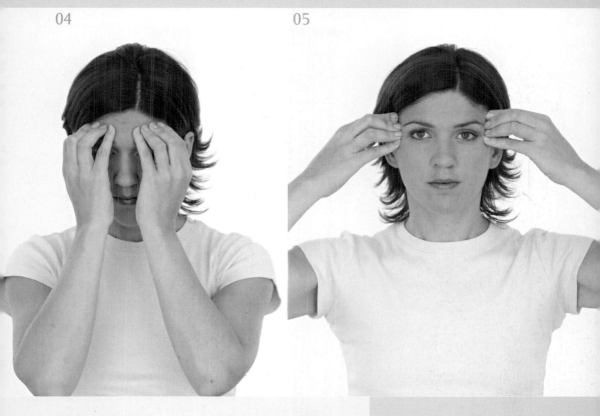

(04) Continue moving your fingers up your forehead and into your hair in 2 cm (¾ in) increments, until you reach the crown of your head. Press and hold in each position for a count of ten.

(05) Place your fingertips in a vertical line at your temples and, again in 2 cm (¾ in) increments, move your fingers back through your hair until they reach the back of your head. Press and hold in each position for a count of ten.

01
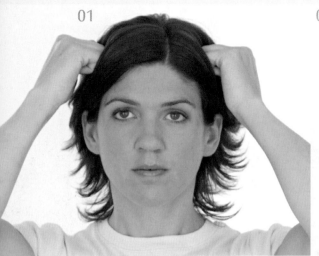

02
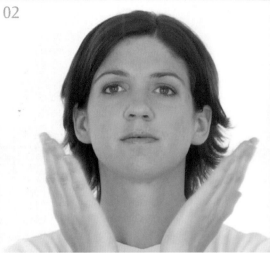

### KNUCKLE RUBBING, SLAPPING, AND EAR PULLING

All these will help to rejuvenate and rebalance your whole system, and wake up your brain! **Do not use ear pulling if you are suffering from earache, ear damage, or infection.**

(01) Knuckle rub briskly all over your head.

(02) With open hands, slap your face briskly all over.

(03) Take hold of the tops of your ears between your index fingertips and thumbs. Pinch around the rim of your ears.

03
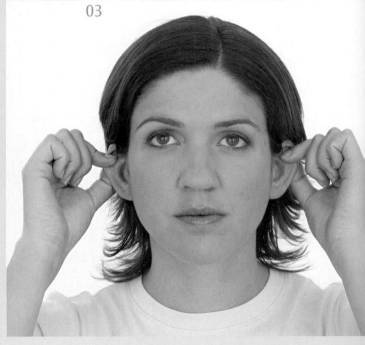

04

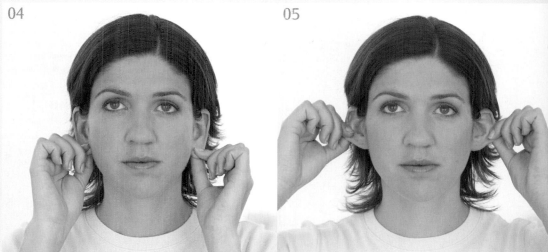

05

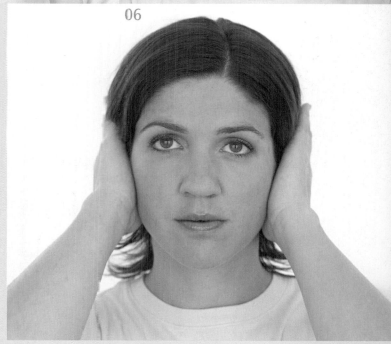

06

*(04) When you reach the earlobes, pull in a downwards direction for a few seconds.*

*(05) Pull your ears out sideways from your head and hold for a few seconds.*

*(06) Place your open hands over your ears and rub briskly for a few seconds.*

# CHAPTER FOUR

# Calming coffee break

No matter what your occupation, working too long without a break creates tension in your back, shoulder, and neck muscles, tired eyes, and slower, more easily irritated mental processes.

Any good boss will encourage you to take a break that includes active exercise. Ideally, you should try to take a brief walk in the fresh air, as a recycled air-conditioned atmosphere is not the best for brain work and active, creative thinking. Throughout the day, try running up and down stairs, and use the washroom that is furthest from your desk.

During your break, a few minutes spent loosening up with head massage, working either on yourself or with a colleague, can make the rest of your day both more enjoyable and more productive.

Many headaches and eyestrains can be aggravated by tight muscles in the upper back and shoulders. These respond very well to any technique that applies a holding pressure. During a break it can be very refreshing to share a back, shoulder, and head massage of this kind with a colleague. No matter where a headache occurs, it is good to work on the whole of your head with massage.

### CANDLE BREATHING

To calm, refresh, and energize your mind and body, sit for a few moments with this visualization and breathing exercise. You could sprinkle a couple of drops of lavender or geranium oil on a tissue and breathe in the vapour while you relax.

During this visualization you will be moving the candle flame through different colours of the spectrum.

If you are tired – start with a white flame and gradually, with each breath, change the colour of the flame through yellow and orange to scarlet.

If you are agitated – move the colour from purple through dark and mid-blue to ice blue.

If you are angry – move the colour from holly green through calm sea green and turquoise to sky blue.

To clear your head – move the colour from sage green through yellow then white to pale pink.

You may like to experiment with other colour journeys, depending on how you feel. Go with whatever feels good.

Close your eyes and imagine a candle in front of you. Throughout, breathe in through your nose and out through your mouth.

Breathe in – take the breath deep down into your hara (lower abdomen).

Breathe out – blow onto the candle to light its flame. See and feel its colour.

Breathe in – take the colour into your body.

Breathe out – blow the colour back into the candle.

Repeat the exercise with this one colour until you can feel its influence and notice yourself changing.

When you are ready, on an out-breath, move the colour on to the next shade.

Repeat until you can feel yourself being moved by the colour, then move on to the next shade.

Continue with the colour-changing cycle for as long as is necessary to revitalize your mind and body.

With a little practice, this exercise will be very effective if done for only a few minutes. **Do not use lavender oil during pregnancy (see page 87).**

# Quick refresher

This meditation and massage sequence quickly frees up any tightness in your body and mind, releasing and refreshing your organizational and creative abilities.

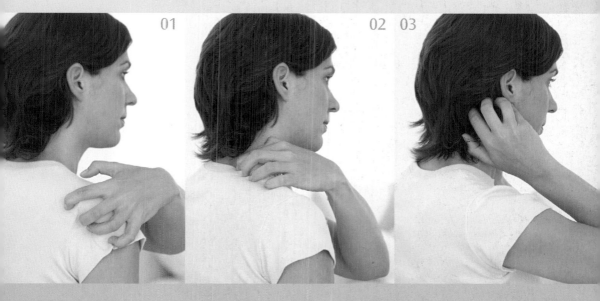

**NECK RUB**
This routine will loosen up any tension across your shoulders and neck.
**Do not work across your shoulders during pregnancy (see page 14).**

(01) Place the fingers of one hand on your opposite

shoulder. With firm pressure, rotate your fingers into your shoulder for a few seconds. The pressure here can cause some pain, but should not be too uncomfortable.

(02) Move your fingers about four finger-widths closer to your neck and repeat, then

move your fingers up onto your neck and repeat.

(03) Move up your neck until your fingers are pressing into the base of your skull and repeat. Change hands and work along your other shoulder and up onto the other side of your neck.

### NECK STRETCHES

*These stretches help to clear long-held tension and stiffness, thereby increasing the flexibility of your neck. They also stretch the muscles, allowing any build-up of toxins to be released.*

*(01) Take hold of the left side of your head with your right hand. Place your left hand with the heel under the right side of your chin. Carefully push on your chin while pulling on the top of your head. Take the twist only as far as is comfortable. Hold for a count of 10–15. Relax and release your head.*

*(02) Bend your head forwards and clasp your hands at the back of your neck. Pull down with your hands while you try to resist the pull by pushing your head up. Hold this position for a count of 10–15. Relax and release your head.*

*(03) Take hold of both sides of your neck as you push your head straight up with your hands. It may be easier for you if you can get a colleague to help with this movement by clasping your*

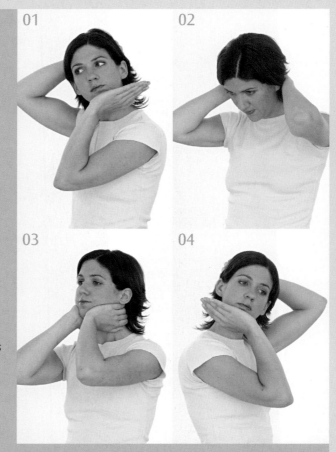

*head in their hands and carefully pulling upwards.*

*(04) Take hold of the right side of your head with your left hand. Place your right hand with the heel under the left side of your chin.*

*Carefully push on your chin with your right hand while pulling on the top of your head with your left. Take the twist only as far as is comfortable. Hold for a count of 10–15. Relax and release your head.*

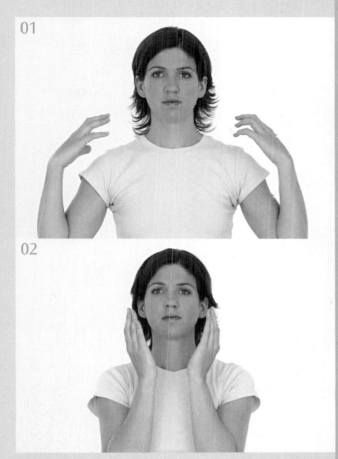

01

02

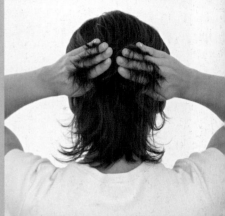

## TAPPING AND SLAPPING
This routine will help to invigorate your facial tissues, improve blood circulation to the surface of the scalp and stimulate the flow of nutrients to the hair roots.

(01) With loose fingers, briskly tap all over your shoulders, neck, and head.

(02) With open hands, slap briskly and firmly all over your face. Take care over your eyes.

## HAIR PULLING
Use these movements to strengthen hair roots, improve circulation in the scalp, rebalance scalp oils, and help to release dry and damaged skin from the scalp.

Run your fingers through the hair over the top of your head, then close them together so that you are holding a good handful of hair in each hand. Pull outwards firmly away from the scalp with the hair under tension. Repeat this until you have pulled through the hair all over your head.

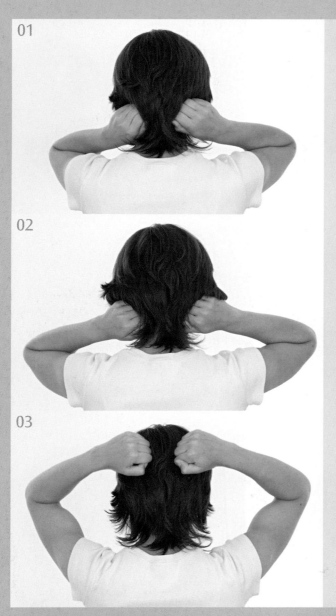

**BACK OF THE HEAD KNUCKLE RUB**

*This technique stimulates your brain, eases tired eyes, aids the circulation of cerebrospinal fluids (which move self-healing messages around the spine and brain), and helps to improve the flexibility of your neck.*

*(01) Close your hands into fists and, starting at the back of your neck on either side of your spine, rub strongly with your knuckles across the back of your neck.*

*(02) Move your fists upwards to the base of your skull and again rub strongly.*

*(03) Move your fists up to the crown of your head and rub strongly again.*

(04) Go back to your neck and position your fists on either side and about 5 cm (2 in) out from your spine. Rub strongly into this area.

(05) Move your fists up to the edge of your skull and again rub strongly. This position may feel a little sensitive, so rub only as hard as feels comfortable.

(06) Move your fists up by about 5 cm (2 in), level with your crown and 3–4 cm (1¼–1½ in) away from the centre on either side. Again rub vigorously.

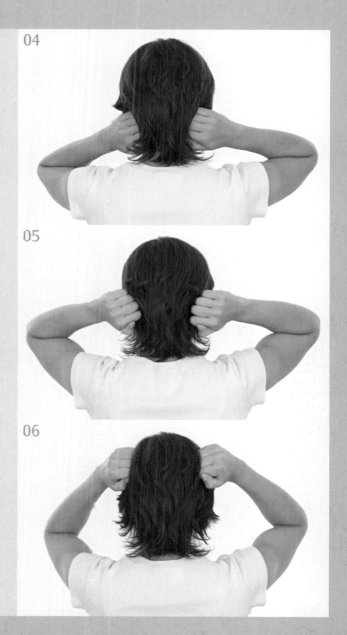

04

05

06

# Headache solutions

There are many types of headache, the most common being caused by stress and tension, particularly around the face, scalp, and back of the neck. Mental turmoil can also be a cause of headaches. Taking time to slow down with a massage and a refreshing breathing and visualization exercise can go a long way towards reducing immediate pain.

## TENSION HEADACHES

These can occur anywhere in your head, face, and neck, and may be caused by clenching your teeth, hunching your shoulders, facial tension, and tightness in the muscles in your scalp. They respond quickly to appropriate massage.

01

### SQUEEZING AND PRESSING

*Stress and tension cause pain in a variety of muscles – this first routine works on your shoulders, neck, and head.*

*(01) Squeeze across one shoulder by working your fingers against the heel of your hand. Repeat on the other shoulder.*

*(02) Bend your head forwards and squeeze up the back of your neck.*

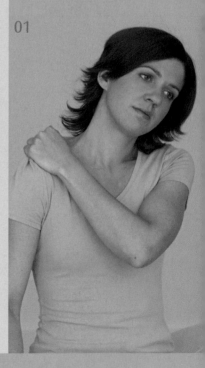

02    03

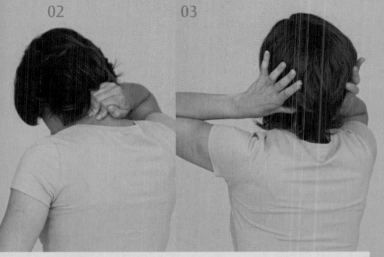

04

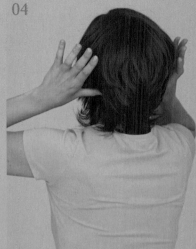

05

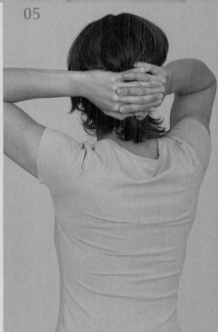

(03) On either side of your spine, just where it meets your head, are two dimpled areas. Place your thumbs in the dimples and lean your head back, so that you are holding the weight of your head on your thumbs. Breathe slowly and deeply. Hold for a count of 20–30. Release and relax.

(04) Move your thumbs out by about two finger widths and again lean your head back onto them for a count of 20–30. Continue moving your thumbs apart by two finger widths each time, rocking your head back and holding

the pressure as above, until you reach your ears.

(05) Place the heels of your hands behind your ears with your fingers towards the back of your head, and clasp your fingers. If you can't reach to interlock your fingers, press into your head with the heels of your hands. Slowly, and with a strong pressure, slide the heels of your hands towards each other until they meet. Move your hands up by a palm's width and repeat. When you reach the crown of your head, continue the action across the top.

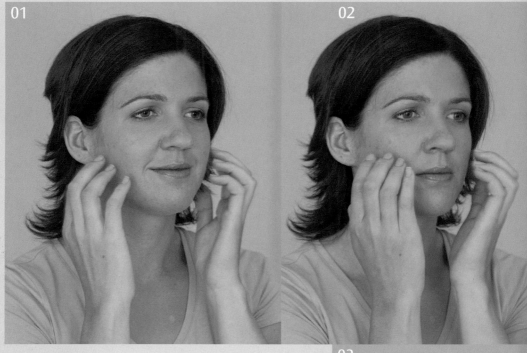

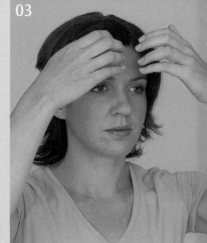

### TAPPING

This is a more focused technique than the tapping described on page 73, and will give a deeper, more specific treatment to release tension and pain.

(01) Starting on either side of your face, level with your jaw, tap with loose fingers in an upwards direction until you reach the hairline.

(02) Return your hands to your jaw, this time on either side of your mouth, and tap upwards again.

(03) Place your fingers in a vertical line just above your nose. Tap out across your forehead towards the temples.

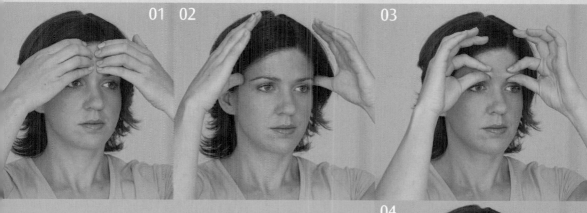

01  02  03

## PRESSURE

There are many areas on your face that can help to release toxins, relax your breathing, tone your system, and reduce tension within the muscles of your face. This sequence will give a general treatment covering many of these areas.

(01) Place your fingers in a vertical line in the centre of your forehead and press with all fingers. Hold for a count of five. Move your fingers outwards by about 2 cm (¾ in) and press again. Repeat until you reach your temples.

(02) Drop your thumbs down into the hollows at the temples and press strongly into this area. Hold for a count of 20.

(03) Pinch with your fingers and thumbs across both of your eyebrows.

(04) Place your fingertips along your cheekbones and press and hold with an upwards, medium pressure for a count of ten. Be careful not to drag downwards.

(05) Smooth the palms of your hands over your face and head in an upwards and outwards direction.

04

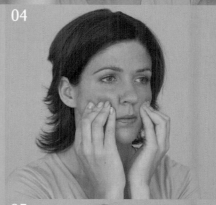

05

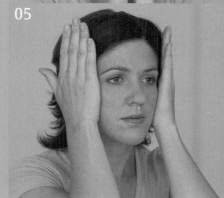

## CLOSING SEQUENCE

*To finish, apply pressure to a variety of points and end with a relaxing hold over your eyes.*

*(01) With your forefinger and thumb, pinch with a medium pressure (or as strong a pressure as is comfortable) on either side of your nose, level with your eyes. Hold for a count of five and release. Repeat this on/off pressure for about a minute.*

*(02) Move your thumbs up to the inner corners of your eyebrows and repeat the on/off pressure as above.*

*(03) Place your elbows on a desk or table. Put the heels of your hands together level with your nose and lean the weight of your head into your hands, with the hollows of your palms covering, but not pressing on, your eyes. Maintaining this position, gently stroke your temples with your thumbs. Stay in this position for as long as you feel is necessary.*

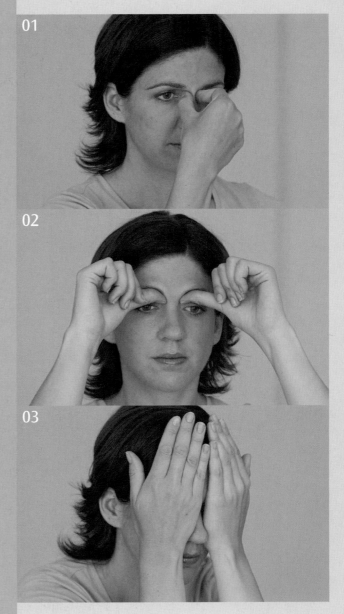

01

02

03

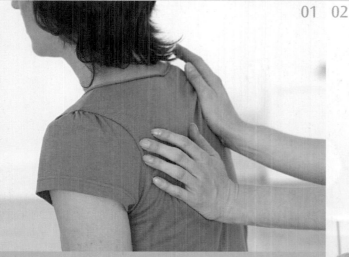

01  02

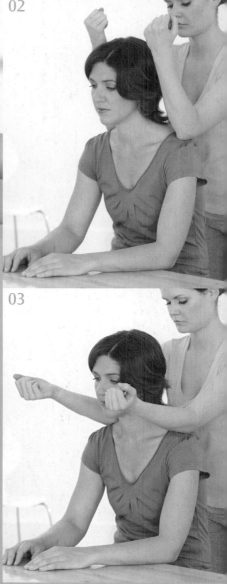

03

## BACK AND SHOULDER MASSAGE WITH A COLLEAGUE

Tension in the upper back, neck, and scalp is often responsible for eyestrain, headaches, and sinus problems. Massaging these areas as well as the face can quickly relieve pain.

(01) Have your partner sit forwards with elbows supported on the desk or the arms of the chair. Massage strongly across your partner's upper back by pressing in the heels of your hands on either side of the spine at the level of the shoulder blades, and then 'walking' your weight from hand to hand up the back to the shoulders. Repeat five to six times.

(02) With your partner sitting upright, place your elbows on the shoulders on either side of the head and close your fists. Lean down and hold for a count of five. **Do not use this technique during pregnancy (see page 14).**

(03) The pressure can be varied by opening and closing the gap between your fists and your shoulders. The wider the gap, the lighter the pressure; the narrower the gap, the stronger and sharper the elbows feel.

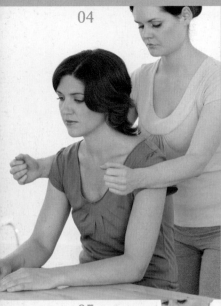

04

*(04) Using your forearms, squeeze inwards at the top of your partner's arms. Run your arms down to the elbows. Repeat three times.*

*(05) Squeeze across the top of your partner's shoulders, working your fingers against the heels of your hands. **Do not use this technique during pregnancy (see page 14).***

*(06) Finish off with a firm, vigorous knuckle rub across the back and shoulders.*

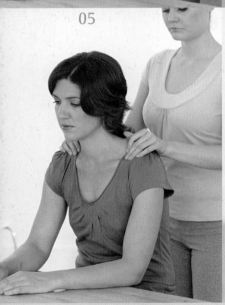

05

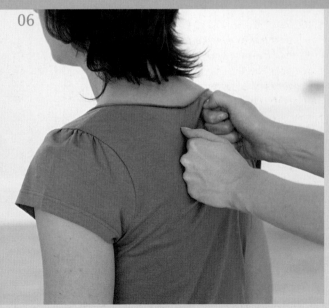

06

## MIGRAINE

Migraine is a more complicated problem than a straightforward headache, as it can be caused more by lifestyle and diet than by your immediate circumstances. It is not really advisable to use massage in the case of migraines. However, if the migraine has passed its peak but is lingering, a light all-over massage can help to move it on, but take care: it could also make you feel very much worse during the migraine's progress.

### COOLING VISUALIZATION

*Place your hands over your eyes and be aware of the space between the palms and your eyes. Breathe slowly and evenly while feeling the energy coming from your palms. Imagine this penetrating your eyes, going deep into your brain, and filling your head with a cool, healing, blue light. Stay in this position until the visual disturbances have cleared.*

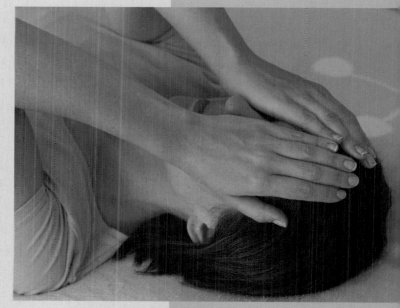

# CHAPTER FIVE

# Time to relax

No matter how sociable and gregarious you may be, spending some time that is just for you, on your own and unwinding in your special space, is one of the most precious gifts you can give yourself.

M editation and visualization are an important part of the releasing process enabling the effects of massage to penetrate both deep within your being and to the outermost edges of your aura. Practising these techniques will connect and unify your being, allowing you to feel whole, strong, energized, and able to take on the challenges of the days ahead.

Go on, be selfish for a while. Enjoy the lightness that you will feel by allowing your problems to take care of themselves. In fact, if there is a problem you are struggling to solve, write it down on a piece of paper before you start your special time. Place the paper face down far away from you, so that you can't see it, and then forget about it. Settle down and enjoy all the freedom and pampering before you. As you finish the session, ways of solving your problem are virtually guaranteed to emerge.

This chapter begins with suggestions for using oils to relax and restore your body and spirit, and free up your mind from the day's concerns. Hair treatments and tonics are also included, which will work with the head massage to enrich and enliven your hair.

# Using oils

Traditionally, the oil used in Indian head massage is coconut oil, which is applied to the hair following massage. Alternatively, you could use essential oils as in aromatherapy, selecting them for their aromatic and therapeutic qualities, and applying them at the start of the massage. You could use a brush to work the oil through your hair, or rub the oil onto your hands and then massage your head, neck, and face. Details of carrier oils and quantities to use are given on page 88.

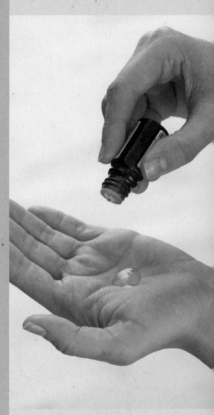

### COCONUT OIL

This traditional oil is solid in the jar, so must be melted in the palm of your hand just before applying to the hair following massage.

Take about 5 ml (1 teaspoon) of the oil and allow it to melt in your hand. Rub it between your palms until it is liquid, then work it through the hair until the whole head is coated. If your hair is long, you may need up to 15 ml (1 tablespoon) of the oil.

Wrap your head in a towel and leave the oil on overnight, then shampoo it out, leaving your hair sleek and glossy.

This treatment is most beneficial when applied every four to six weeks, depending on hair type: dry hair will need a four-week interval, normal hair six weeks. If your hair is greasy, use massage only, which will help to regulate the flow of nutrients and oils to the surface of the scalp.

## OTHER OILS
**Chamomile** Flower. Very good for fair to blond hair. Encourages calmness, control, and easy acceptance.
**Citrus** Leaf/flower. Clears the head and lifts the spirits.
**Cedarwood** Wood. Decongestant and calming. Also antiviral and antibacterial, which makes it very good for any head infections (see hair tonic recipe on page 89).
**Eucalyptus** Leaf. Encourages optimism, openness, and freedom.
**Frankincense** Wood. Brings spiritual liberation and tranquil contemplation.
**Geranium** Leaf. Opens up feelings of security, receptivity, and intimacy.
**Lavender** Flower. An excellent general-purpose oil which brings feelings of calm composure and easy self-expression. It is very healing as it is antiviral and antibiotic.
**Peppermint** Leaf. Good for headaches and relieves mental cloudiness.
**Rosemary** Flower. As well as being antiviral, this oil deepens awareness of identity, dedication, and destiny, and rebalances the body and mind.
**Sandalwood** Wood. Soothing and calming.
**Tea tree** Leaf. Good for mental strength, resistance, and confidence. It is very healing as it is antiviral and antibiotic.
**White Pine** Leaf/wood. Creates a feeling of space and openness.
**Vetiver** Wood/root. Very nourishing. Restores and reconnects well-being.
**Ylang-ylang** Leaf. Relaxing. Encourages a sensual zing and euphoria.

*TAKE CARE*
*Citrus, lavender, rosemary* Do not use these oils during pregnancy or in cases of high blood pressure.
*Eucalyptus* Do not use where there are kidney problems.
*Peppermint* Do not use in the bath as it may sting sensitive areas.

*The oils suggested for use here are very safe. However, any substance can cause a reaction in a small minority of people. Therefore, if you have not used an oil before, it is advisable to do a skin test on the inside of your wrist. Leave for 24 hours – if the skin shows any sign of reddening or irritation, do not use the oil.*

## PREPARATION OF OILS

For most applications, dilute 5 drops essential oil in 20 ml (4 teaspoons) carrier oil (such as olive, sweet almond, coconut, or sesame). If you are using more than one essential oil, the total amount should not exceed 5 drops per 20 ml (4 teaspoons) carrier oil.

As a general rule, when making up your own mixtures it is better to choose no more than two oils: one flower/leaf extraction and one wood/root extraction. Otherwise, the oils may 'fight' with each other. Recipes for specific treatments are given below.

## APPLICATION OF OILS

The massage oils may be used on your arms, shoulders, and neck as in aromatherapy treatments by coating your hands regularly with about 5 ml (1 teaspoon) of the mixture. Stroke your oiled hands over the area to be massaged with long, flowing movements to distribute the oil, before going into the deeper movements. Avoid using the oils on your face as you may accidentally get some in your eyes.

You can use the oils in your hair in a similar manner by recoating your hands regularly with the mixture during the head massage sequence. Leave the oil in your hair for about 24 hours before washing. *Remember, do not use citrus, lavender, or rosemary oils during pregnancy (see page 87).*

## Normal/dry hair

Dilute 5 drops of rosemary, lavender, or geranium oil in 20 ml (4 teaspoons) carrier oil such as almond or coconut.

### Greasy hair/dandruff
Dilute 5 drops of rosemary or lavender oil in 20 ml
(4 teaspoons) sweet almond oil.

### Thinning hair
Dilute 5 drops of rosemary, lavender, geranium,
or ylang-ylang oil in 20 ml (4 teaspoons) sesame or
olive oil.

### Hair tonic
This tonic is a good general treatment for out-of-
condition hair that is dull and lacks vitality

*3 drops rosemary oil*
*3 drops ylang-ylang oil*
*2 drops cedarwood oil*
*5 ml (1 teaspoon) vodka*
*30 ml (2 tablespoons) orange flower water*

Add the rosemary or lavender, ylang-ylang, and
cedarwood oils to the vodka and stir thoroughly.
Mix with the orange flower water. Massage through
your hair and leave on for 24 hours before
shampooing it out.

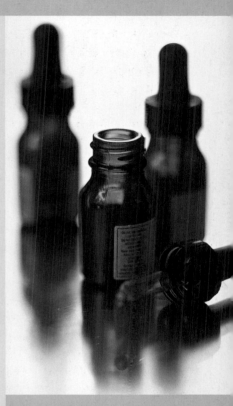

# Setting the scene

Even if you are working on yourself, you will find that the treatment will be much more effective, enjoyable, and relaxing if you take the time to prepare your surroundings for a pampering and rejuvenating session.

- Make sure the room is warm enough to keep out the winter chill or cool enough if you are at the end of a long, hot, and exhausting day.
- If it is still daylight, close the curtains and use soft candlelight, making sure you have enough ventilation as candle flames can remove a lot of oxygen from the surrounding air.
- You may like to burn incense or essential oil in a vaporizer and have some gentle music playing.
- If you are going to enjoy a scented bath, it is a good idea to do this *before* you use any head massage – this is so relaxing, you could fall asleep in the bath!
- Finally, you may like to make yourself comfortable on a duvet and/or pile of cushions on the floor while you massage, so that afterwards you can curl up and sleep away all your tensions.

**AURA-CLEANSING VISUALIZATION**

*Cleansing your aura helps you to feel clear, pure, and at one with the universal energies. You may feel lighter and cooler, more receptive to healing, freer, and more open to creative ideas – the perfect start to your relaxation session.*

*Sit or stand in a comfortable position and close your eyes. Throughout, breathe in through your nose and out through your mouth.*

*Take a breath and feel the air going right down to your feet.*
  *Breathe out – pull the air up from your feet and out through the top of your head. Repeat for five breaths.*
  *Breathe in – visualize the air glowing as it enters your body, right down to your feet. Hold the breath while you observe your body as if from a short distance away. Notice any variations in the aura around it. Are there any dark, muddy patches or cloudy areas?*

*Breathe out – allow these dark, muddy, or cloudy areas to dissolve and move out of your body and aura with the out-breath. Visualize the muddiness slipping away, far away, out into the universe. Repeat this clearing breath for five to six breaths.*

*Breathe in – visualize a bright white sheet stretched out beneath you.*

*Breathe out – see and feel the white sheet moving up through your body and aura, gathering all the remaining muddiness from your being. Visualize the sheet carrying all the negative energy and disappearing far out into the universe.*

*Breathe in – again observe your body and aura as if from a short distance away. If there are any remaining cloudy areas, repeat the sweep with the white sheet.*

*Allow your breathing to return to normal and open your eyes. Take a moment to enjoy the feelings of lightness and clarity.*

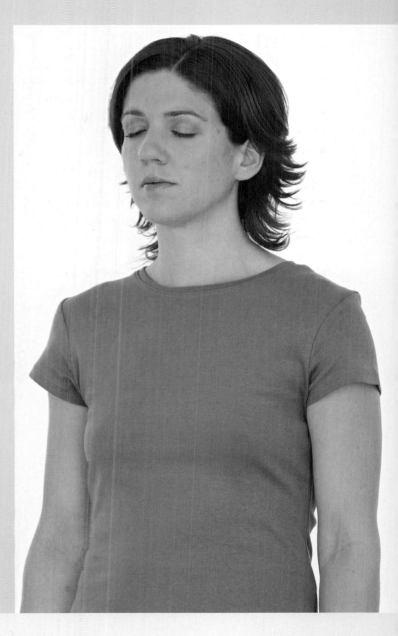

# The massages

Now start your massage sequence. Move slowly and with intention. Focus on every movement of your muscles. Make every movement deliberate, smooth, and flowing. Breathe slowly and evenly throughout the whole treatment.

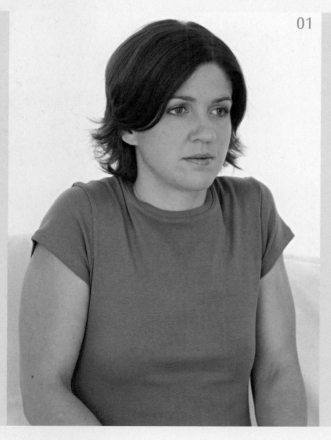

01

*BACK AND SHOULDER RELEASE*
*This is more of an exercise than a massage. It helps to free up any stiffness in your arms and shoulders, and makes it easier to reach those out-of-the-way places on your head, neck, and shoulders.*

*(01) Sit or stand in a comfortable position. Lift your shoulders up to your ears and hold for a count of ten. Relax. Repeat four to five times, after the first couple of times allowing your shoulders to drop suddenly rather than slide down. This releases any tension that could still be held within your muscles if you release your shoulders slowly.*

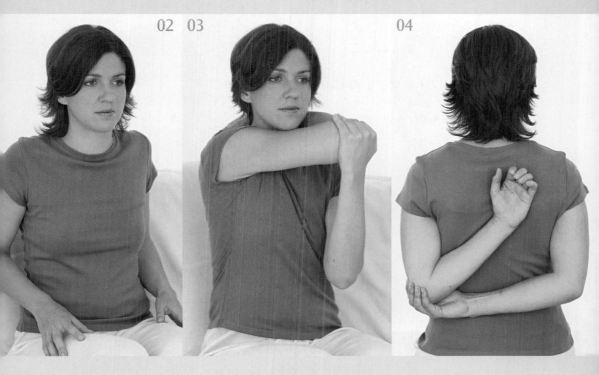

02    03                          04

(02) Rotate your shoulders in a forwards direction four to five times. Then rotate in a backwards direction four to five times.

(03) Place your right hand over your left shoulder. Place your left hand under your right elbow and ease your right arm further over your left shoulder. Hold for a count of ten. Repeat the stretch on your left arm.

(04) Place your left arm behind your back and try to reach up your back with your hand. Place your right arm behind your back and grasp your left elbow with your right hand and pull your arm further across so that you are able to stretch higher up your back. Hold for a count of ten. Repeat the stretch on your right arm.

Relax, and shrug your shoulders a few times. Your back and shoulder muscles should now feel much looser and freer.

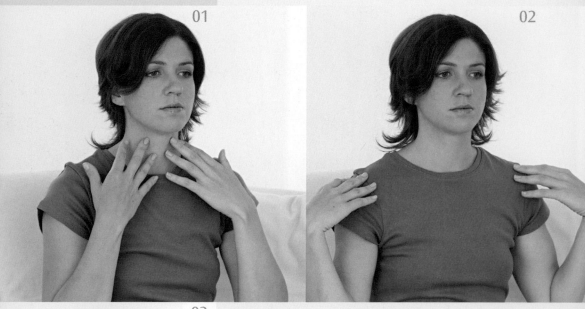

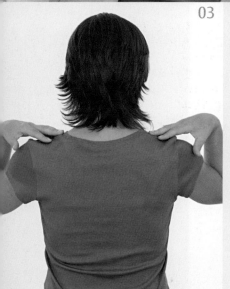

### STROKING

On the in-breath you should stroke down and on the out-breath you should hold the end position. This regulates the rhythm of the stroke and ensures a deeper relaxation during the massage.

(01) Start with both hands on the top of your head. Stroke down your face and throat three to four times.

(02) Go back to the top of your head and stroke down either side of your head and across your shoulders three to four times.

(03) Place your hands on the back of your head, level with the crown, and stroke down the back of your head and neck and across your shoulders three to four times.

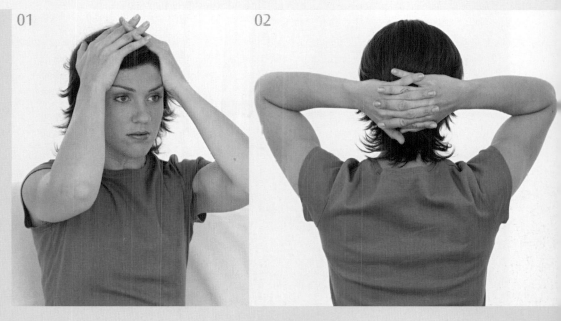

01

02

### GENTLE SQUEEZING

This routine helps to release tension and toxin build-up within the muscles. While you are working through it, remember to breathe slowly and rhythmically.

(01) Sit or stand in a comfortable position. Interlock your fingers and place the heels of your hands just above your temples. With an upwards pressure, squeeze the heels of your hands together, sliding upwards towards the top of your head. Move your hands backwards by about 8 cm (3¼ in) – they should now be just above your ears. Squeeze upwards as before.

(02) Move your hands back again by 8 cm (3¼ in), so that the heels of your hands are just below the crown of your head. Squeeze upwards as before. Place the heels of your hands just behind your ears with the fingers pointing backwards. Squeeze with the heels of your hands as before, moving towards the back of your head.

03

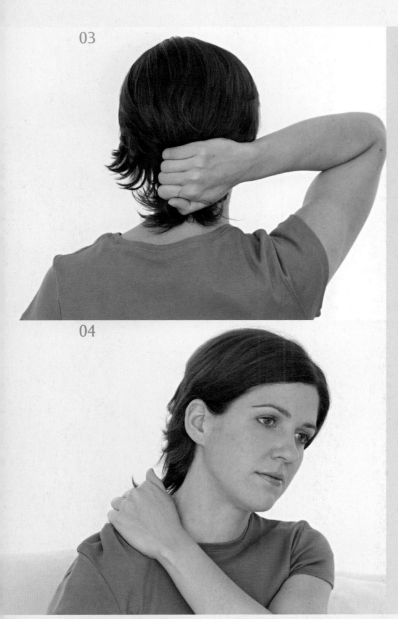

04

(03) With one hand, grasp the back of your neck, just where it joins your head. Squeeze your fingers towards the palm of your hand while pulling your whole hand backwards. Drop your hand by about 6 cm (2½ in) to the base of the neck and squeeze again.

(04) With your left hand on your right shoulder at the base of your neck, squeeze in an upwards direction, moving your fingers firmly towards the heel of your hand. The top of your shoulders may feel tender and painful – this is normal. Move your hand along your shoulder by about 8 cm (3¼ in) and squeeze. Repeat until you reach the shoulder bone. **Do not use this technique if you are pregnant (see page 14).**

05

06

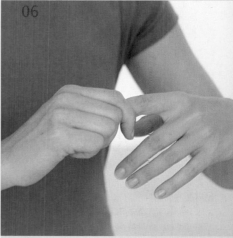

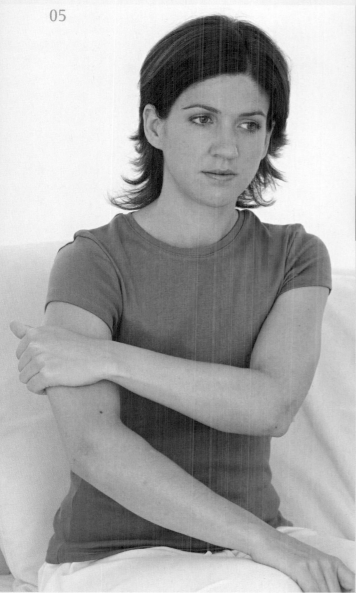

(05) Move down to the top of your arm and continue the squeezing in the same way all along your arm. Repeat the squeezing along your left shoulder, arm, and hand.

(06) To finish, squeeze and shake your fingers.

01                                    02  03

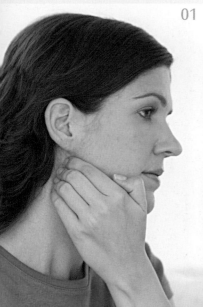 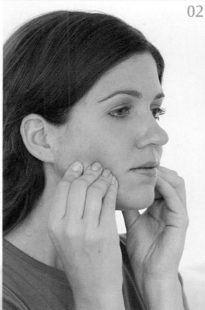 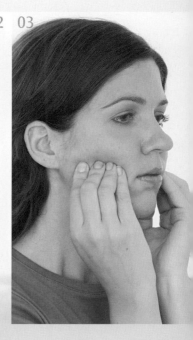

### PRESSURE

With this routine, hold the pressure for two slow breaths in each position. When using pressure on your face, be careful not to drag the skin and muscles in a downwards direction – the pressure should always be in a horizontal or slightly upwards direction. This entire sequence will stimulate areas that help to rebalance and tone your whole system.

(01) Place the fingers of your left hand in a vertical line on your neck just below your right ear and press inwards. Move your fingers about 2 cm (¾ in) forwards and repeat. Repeat this press-and-release routine until you have reached the centre front of your throat, then change hands and repeat over the left side of your neck.

(02) With your thumbs hooked under your jaw in front of your ears and your fingers resting just above your jawline, press inwards and hold. Repeat the pressure at 2 cm (¾ in) intervals along your jaw until your fingers meet in the middle of your chin.

(03) With the fingers of each hand in a horizontal position on either side of your face at jaw level, press and hold. Move 2 cm (¾ in) upwards and repeat. Continue moving up at 2 cm (¾ in) intervals until you reach your hairline.

01

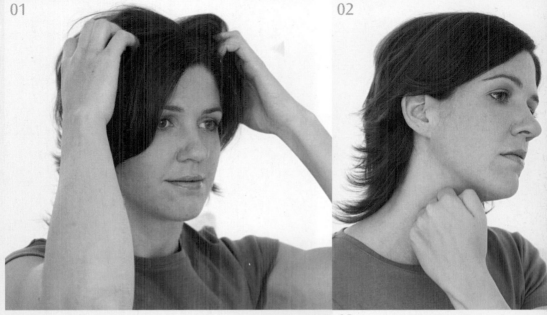

02

### SCRATCHING, KNUCKLE RUBBING, AND ROTATIONS

These are invigorating techniques which will help to improve circulation. This both nourishes your brain and stimulates a good flow of nutrients to the surface of your scalp, helping to improve the condition of your hair and loosen up tight muscles.

(01) Scratch lightly and vigorously all over your head.

(02) Clench your fists and rub your knuckles all over your head, neck, and shoulders.

(03) Hold your hands in a claw shape and press firmly into your scalp with strong fingers. Move your fingers in small rotations all over your scalp and neck.

03

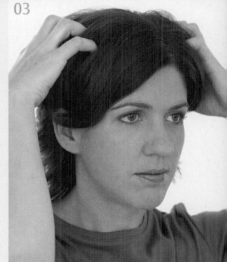

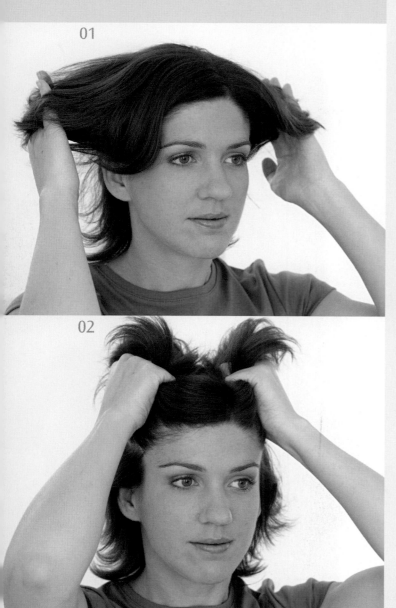

## HAIR PULLING AND SHAKING

The following techniques help to strengthen the hair roots and to reduce tension within your scalp.

(01) Hold your hands with open fingers and slide them deep into your hair. Close your fingers and hold firmly while pulling away from your head in a sideways direction, allowing your hair to run through your fingers under tension. Repeat until you have covered the whole of your head.

(02) Slide your fingers into your hair as before, but this time grasp your hair firmly and shake handfuls of it back and forth, moving the scalp a little.

## EAR PINCHING AND RUBBING

*These actions stimulate the areas of your ears that work to rebalance the energy within your body, helping to maintain good health. **Do not use ear pinching if you are suffering from earache, ear damage, or infection.***

*(01) Take hold of the tops of your ears between your index fingertips and thumbs. Pinch strongly and massage your ears for a few moments. Move back along the outer ridge of your ears by about 2 cm (¾ in) and repeat.*

*(02) When you reach the earlobes, pull in a downwards direction for a few seconds.*

01
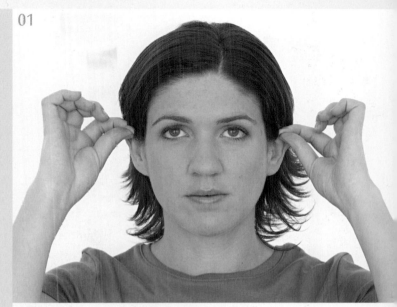

02
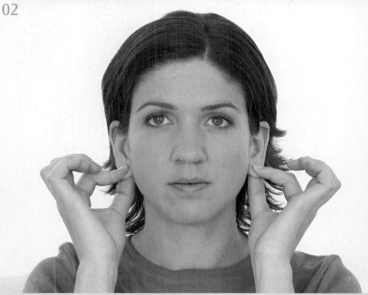

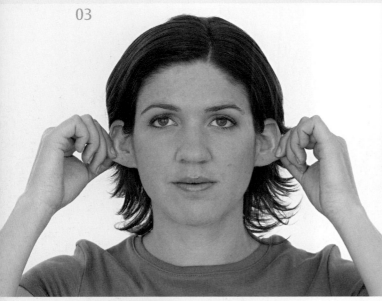

03

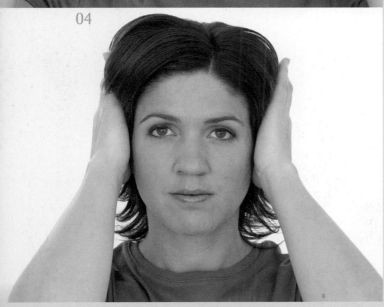

04

*(03) Pull your ears out sideways from your head and hold for a few seconds. By now your ears may be rather hot and red as the blood flow to them increases.*

*(04) Place your open hands over your ears and rub briskly for a few seconds. Hold your palms over your ears for a few moments to allow the muscles to relax.*

05

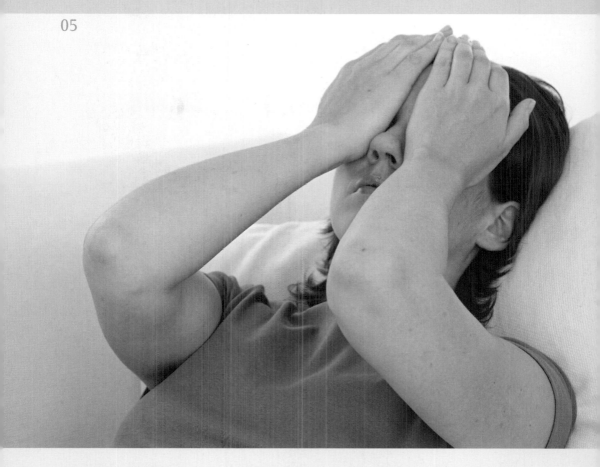

### FINAL RELAXING POSE

When you feel the warmth from this routine building, imagine this feeling moving right through your body and down to your toes. Stay with this feeling for as long as you like – it is incredibly refreshing and healing.

(05) End the session by lying down on your back, placing the palms of your hands gently over your eyes, and relaxing. Feel the warmth of your hands penetrating deep into your eyes. After a few minutes, place your hands gently over your ears. Relax and feel the warmth of your hands penetrating deep into your ears.

# CHAPTER SIX

# The whole works

This chapter combines all the techniques to provide a shared experience for you and your partner that will enrich your lives. It suggests a massage sequence that you can follow until you feel you can work instinctively wherever and in whatever way the massage is needed.

Traditionally, Indian head massage starts with loosening up the back, then moving up into the shoulders, neck, and scalp, finishing with a gentle face massage. However, you may feel you wish to start by working on your partner's face to relax and connect more intimately. Next, move into the hair and over the head, down onto the neck and shoulders, and then onto the back. In this way, a deeper connection is made than would be acceptable for the relationship between a therapist and client, but one that is entirely appropriate for a closer relationship between partners. Go with your instincts and follow your intuition: use this book as a guide, but be free and creative.

Whichever sequence you choose, it is important to work in a way that achieves a smooth flow of movement. You should complete all the work on one part of the head, neck, or shoulders before moving onto a different area, so as to produce a feeling of continuity and rhythm. This will give your partner confidence in your technique and enable them to relax completely in your hands.

# Creating the right atmosphere

For you and your partner to gain the most benefit from your shared massage, it is important to create a relaxing atmosphere that excludes all worldly interferences. The following aspects all combine to make the whole experience enjoyable, healing, refreshing, re-energizing, and relaxing.

**LOW LIGHTING**
During daylight hours simply draw the curtains so that a fine strip of light enters the room, just enough to enable you to see what you are doing. After dark you could use candles, but not too many as they consume oxygen and this can be stifling.

Even better are salt lamps. These are made from solid salt crystals of various sizes, which have been drilled out in the centre and a lamp inserted. The crystals come in yellow, red, orange, and white, providing a wonderful glow that enhances the healing of your session. Another advantage of these lamps is that they ionize the atmosphere and provide a positive charge to the energy in the room, which is very beneficial to your health.

**GOOD VENTILATION**
This is important, as you may feel breathless and overheated after a while, particularly during a long session when you and your partner are breathing the same air, or you are using candles that devour the oxygen. Good ventilation is the single most important thing to consider, as energy flow can feel overpowering in an enclosed atmosphere.

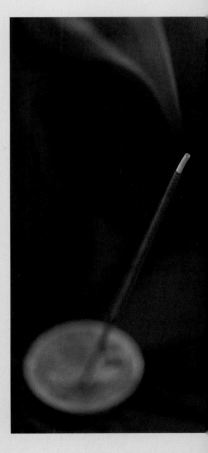

## HARMONIC BLENDING

Music can relax, excite, disturb, ignite memories, and evoke emotions. It is important that you choose the right music for both of your moods – music that sounds relaxing and peaceful to one person can be boring or irritating for another. Choose the music together; if there is disagreement, it is better to use the choice of the receiver than that of the giver. When it is time to change places, the music can also be changed.

## UPLIFTING AROMAS

Like sounds, scents are very evocative. If you are going to burn incense or use essential oils, choose them together. If you feel your partner would benefit from a particular oil, do check that they like the smell before using it, as otherwise it could disrupt the whole session.

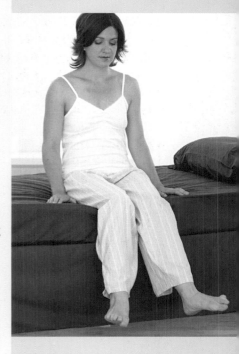

### CLOTHING

*Keep everything free and easy. Wear loose, comfortable clothing, and preferably no shoes. Remove any watches, jewellery, hairbands, or ornaments before you start. This is easy to forget but could create an unwanted interruption if you need to stop partway through the massage to untangle a snagged necklace or clip.*

# Setting the scene

Good, positive energy is important to the atmosphere of a relaxing and healing session. This is particularly important if there has been an emotional disturbance, such as an argument, in the room, even if it happened days or weeks previously.

***CLEARING THE ENERGY***
*Open a window or door to ensure a free flow of energy. During the clearing process, imagine light, positive energy coming into the room and stagnant energy flowing out through the window or door. You can use a singing bowl, a small bell, a gong, or a drum to start the clearing.*

*Starting from the door of the room, you (or your partner) should move in a clockwise direction around the edge, sounding the bowl, (bell, gong, or drum) towards each wall and into each corner of the room.*
 *Work over the same path with burning herbs or incense – sage or frankincense would be a good choice (although sage should not be used during pregnancy).*
 *Shine a candle into the room's nooks and crannies.*

 *With you and your partner standing in the centre of the room, imagine that you are both in the centre of a bubble of light. Visualize this light moving outwards to the walls of the room and filling the whole space with a clear, white light. If there are any worries or cares left over from the day, see them dissolving*

*in the light. Feel and enjoy each other's presence.*
 *You are now beginning to be in tune, and connecting with your partner will progress smoothly.*

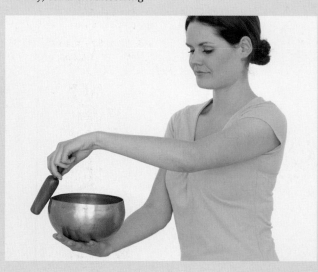

# Connecting with your partner

Connecting can take the form of a shared visualization, or can be done simply by laying your hands on your partner's shoulders, then forehead and base of the skull, then either side of the head, while synchronizing your breathing with your partner's. This enables you both to connect with the free-flowing energy passing between you.

If you wish to connect using a visualization, try the one given below. Alternatively, you can use any of the visualizations on pages 38–41.

### WATERFALL VISUALIZATION

*Sit or stand in a comfortable position with your partner, facing each other. Take your partner's left hand in your right hand and place it over your heart chakra, covering the hand with yours. Do the same with your left hand over your partner's heart chakra and their right hand covering your left. Close your eyes and breathe together for a few moments. Throughout the visualization, breathe in through your nose and out through your mouth.*

*Breathe in – visualize a fall of silver water flowing over and through you both.*

*Breathe out – imagine this silver waterfall washing away all your negative thoughts and emotions.*

*Breathe in – see clear silver water filling you both with a light, joyful energy.*

*Continue this visualization until you can feel the water from the silver waterfall filling your entire being.*

*Without breaking the connection you have made, proceed with the head massage. Move slowly and lightly, allowing your feelings to dictate the massage.*

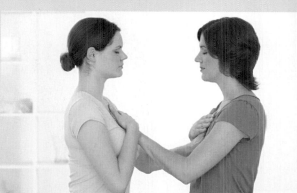

# The massages

The sequence presented here moves the massage from the back and shoulders, up into the neck and onto the head, culminating in a light face and ear massage to complete. Remember that you can perform the various routines in a different order if you and your partner prefer (see pages 106–107).

## BACK AND SHOULDER WORK

Daily irritations, worries, stress, and tension all accumulate in the muscles of your upper back, shoulders, and neck. If these negative influences are allowed to build up unchecked, they will eventually start to create ill-health. The strokes in this and the next section (Neck work, pages 122–124) will enable both you and your partner to release all that the day has thrown at you.

## *BACK LOOSENING*

*This technique will warm up and loosen the muscles of the upper back and shoulders ready for the stronger and deeper work.*

*(01) Support your partner with one arm across the upper chest. With the heel of your other hand, rub briskly and firmly in small, circular movements all over your partner's upper back.*

*(02) A gentler, but still warming, back rub can be applied using the flat palm of your hand.*

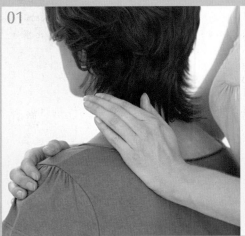

01

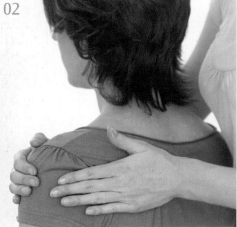

02

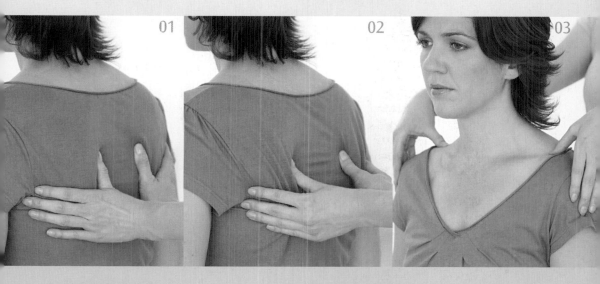

**THUMB PRESSURE**
This is a deep pressure
technique that will move
rapidly through knotted
tension in muscles.

(01) With your partner
leaning forwards slightly,
place your hands with the
heels on either side of the
spine, just below the
shoulder blades. Your
thumbs should be pointing
upwards and your fingers
reaching out towards your
partner's sides. Using a firm
pressure, hold the tips of
your fingers in position while
moving your thumbs towards
your fingers, sliding strongly
through the muscles until
thumbs and fingers touch.
You can lift the heels of your
hands away from the body,
but keep a strong contact
with your fingers and
thumbs. Repeat the
movement three times
in this position.

(02) Keeping your hands at
the same level, hold your
thumbs in position and, with
a strong pressure, draw your
fingers back towards your
thumbs. Repeat three times.

Move your hands upwards
by about 10 cm (4 in) and
repeat the pushing and
pulling stroke. Continue
until you reach the top of
your partner's shoulders,
where you should place your
fingertips on the top of each
arm and your thumbs close
to either side of your
partner's neck.

(03) Slide your thumbs
strongly along the top of
your partner's shoulders,
three times. **Do not use this
technique during pregnancy
(see page 14).**

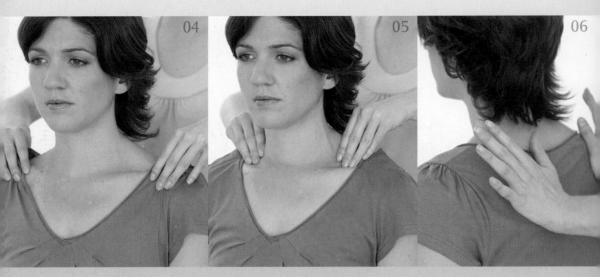

04

05

06

*(04) With your fingers positioned on the front of your partner's shoulders near the tops of the arms and working across the tops of the shoulders, slide across the shoulders with your thumbs three times.* **Do not use this technique during pregnancy (see page 14).**

*(05) Place your thumbs on your partner's back with your fingers to the front of the* shoulders and, with a strong pressure, pull your fingers backwards towards your thumbs, three times. **Do not use this technique during pregnancy (see page 14).**

*Move your hands 5 cm (2 in) closer to your partner's neck and repeat – working your thumbs towards your fingers three times, then working your fingers towards your thumbs three times.*

*Keep the pressure strong and constant.* **Do not use this technique during pregnancy (see page 14).** *Move your hands again, 5 cm (2 in) closer to your partner's neck, and repeat. You should now be at the base of the neck.*

*(06) Rub briskly across your partner's upper back and shoulders with the heels of your hands.*

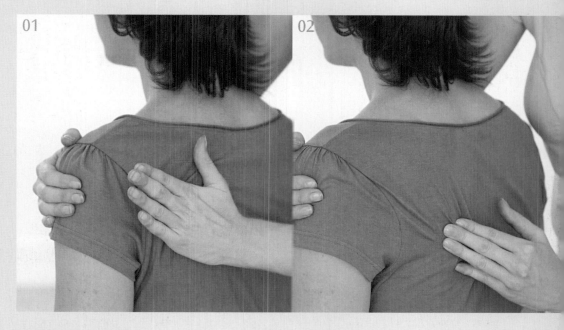

**HEEL OF HAND SLIDE**
*This routine provides a broad, sliding pressure in a back-and-forth action that works strongly into the muscle tissues.*

*(01) Support your partner with one arm across the upper chest. Place the heel of your other hand close to the spine just below the shoulder blades and slide it across your partner's back towards the side, keeping the pressure strong and even.*

*(02) Roll the pressure along your hand to the fingers and slide back strongly, pulling the muscles towards your partner's spine. Repeat this three times. Move your hand upwards by about 10 cm (4 in) and repeat the whole movement. Continue moving your hand upwards, repeating the movement until you reach the base of the neck. Then, change hands and work across the other side of your partner's back.*

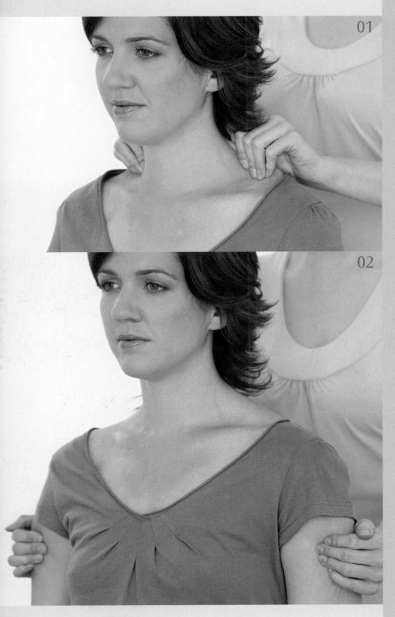

01

02

### SHOULDER AND ARM SQUEEZE

*This is a deep releasing technique that loosens up the whole of the shoulder area.*

*(01) Place your hands on your partner's shoulders, on either side of the neck. Firmly grasp the flesh and pull upwards. Hold this position for a count of five and release. Move your hands outwards by about 5 cm (2 in) and repeat the flesh pull.*

*(02) Again move your hands outwards, to the tops of your partner's arms. Grasp and pull the muscle outwards in a sideways direction. Hold for a count of five and release. Repeat the grasping and pulling at 5 cm (2 in) intervals all the way down your partner's arms.*

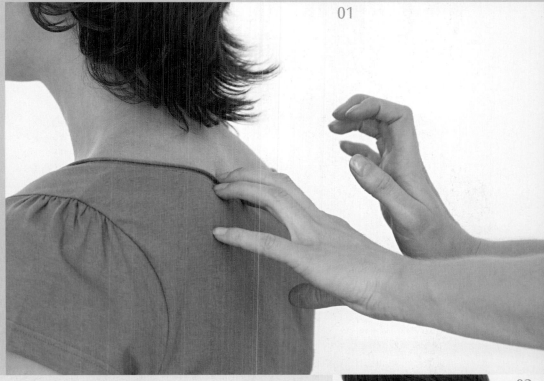

01

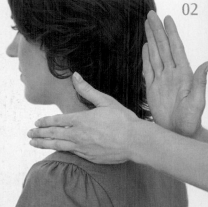

02

### TAPPING AND HACKING
*These percussive strokes help to tone and invigorate muscles in the upper back and shoulders.*

*(01) Holding your fingers bent and relaxed, tap all over your partner's upper back and shoulders in a loose, rhythmical manner.*

*(02) Keeping your hands straight and firm, rapidly hack all over your partner's upper back and shoulders. You can continue this tapping and hacking down the arms if you wish.*

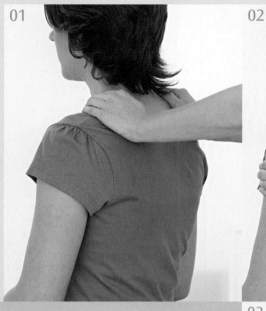

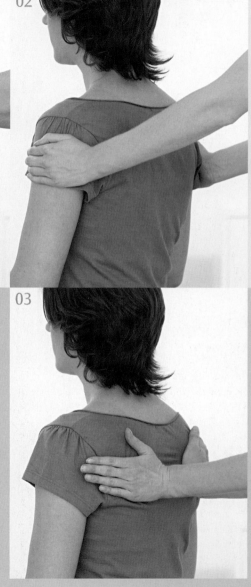

### PRESSURE SLIDE
You can use your hands or your forearms for this routine.

(01) Start with your hands (or forearms) at the base of your partner's neck.

(02) Slide with a firm, steady pressure across the shoulders and down the arms.

(03) Move your hands (or forearms) down to your partner's shoulder blades and slide across the back.

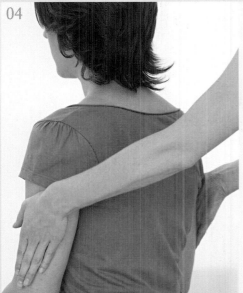

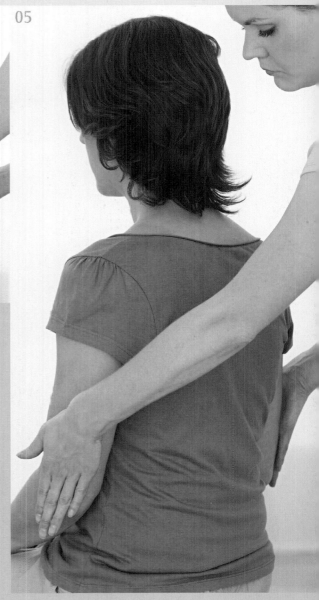

*(04) Place your hands on the tops of your partner's arms. By pushing with the heels of your hands, slide down the sides of their arms to the elbows, maintaining a strong, even pressure.*

*(05) Move your hands back to the tops of your partner's arms and repeat, this time sliding down the backs of your partner's arms.*

## TWO-HAND SQUEEZE

*This technique lifts and releases muscles, helping to remove waste matter and toxins from the tissues and relax any deeply held tension in the shoulders.*

*(01) Stand to one side of your partner. Interlock your fingers and place the heels of your hands on either side of your partner's shoulder, close to the neck. Squeeze the heels of your hands together while at the same time sliding your hands upwards, so that you are pulling the muscles away from the shoulder bone. Move your hands to the centre of the shoulder and repeat the technique.*

*(02) Move your hands to the top of your partner's arm and repeat the squeeze and pull. Move your hands down by about 10 cm (4 in) and repeat. Continue the squeezing until you reach the elbow.*

*Now move to the other side of your partner and repeat the routine.*

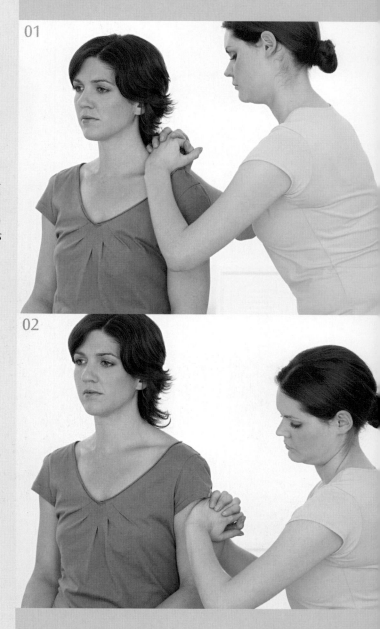

01

02

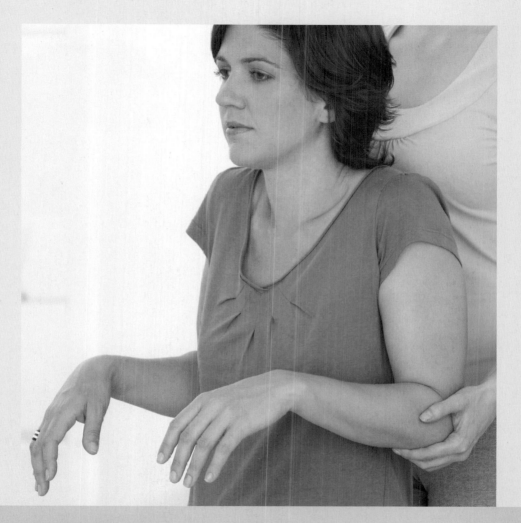

**SHOULDER SHRUGGING**
This exercise will help to free up any stiffness in the shoulder joint.

Stand behind your partner and take hold of the elbows with your hands. Lift directly upwards as far as your partner finds comfortable. Hold for a count of three, then quickly release. Repeat this three to five times.

## NECK WORK

Releasing your partner's neck will help to ease eyestrain and many tension headaches. The massages should be done as a continuous routine, flowing from one stroke to the next.

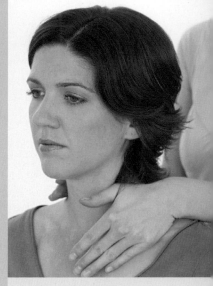

### PULLING

*This technique helps to release any tightness and rigidity within the neck and back of the scalp.*

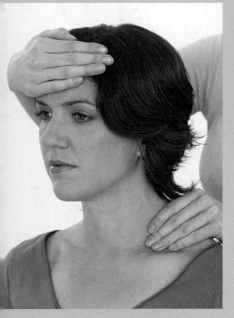

*Support your partner's forehead with one hand. Place the other hand with your thumb about 4 cm (1½ in) to one side of the spine at the back of the neck close to the base, and your fingers about 4 cm (1½ in) to the other side of the spine on the neck. Grasp the flesh of the neck in a clamping movement and pull it away from the bone. Allow your fingers and thumb to slide backwards away from the neck until you have released all the flesh.*

*Move your hand up the neck by about 5 cm (2 in) and repeat the movement. Move up by another 5 cm (2 in) and repeat.*
  *Return to the original position and repeat the whole sequence twice more.*

### STROKING

*This is an excellent warm-up for your partner's neck.*

*Place your hands on either side of the base of the neck and, by working one hand after the other, stroke your hands over towards the throat several times.*

*Move your hands upwards by about 5 cm (2 in) and repeat the stroke towards the throat. You should feel your partner's neck relax and begin to move slightly with the rhythm of your hands.*

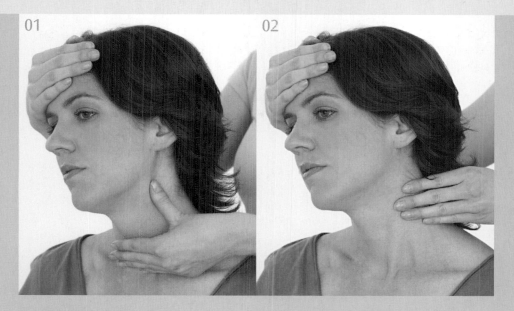

### ALTERNATE FINGERS AND THUMBS

This stroke helps to release any build-up of waste matter and toxins in the muscles of the neck.

*(01) Support your partner's forehead with one hand. Using this hand, lean the head slightly to the side, away from you. Place the thumb of your other hand up close to the hairline, on the near side of the spine. Working along the elongated side of the neck and using a firm pressure, push your thumb from the back to the front of the neck.*

*(02) Place your fingers in the final position of your thumb and pull backwards, still maintaining a firm pressure.*

*Move your fingers down by about 3 cm (1¼ in) and repeat the stroke. Move your fingers down again to the base of the neck and repeat once more. Change hands and work the other side of the neck in the same way.*

01

02

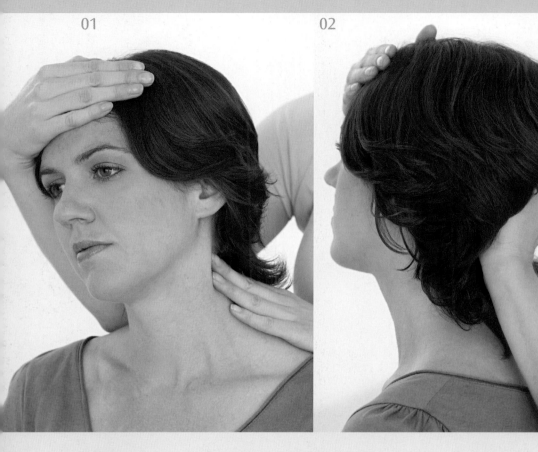

### FRICTION
This technique will loosen up all of the muscles in the back of the neck, freeing up neck movement.

(01) Support your partner's forehead with one hand. Tilt the head forwards slightly and, using the fingers of your other hand, briskly and firmly rub all across the back of your partner's neck with small circular movements.

(02) Use your supporting hand to tilt your partner's head backwards slightly, so that pressure is kept constant between your hands. Using the heel of your other hand and small circular movements, rub firmly into the base of the skull.

## HEAD WORK

After removing all tension within your partner's upper back, shoulders, and neck comes the final liberation. Working on your partner's head moves the energy upwards and outwards, releasing every last scrap of stress, aches, pains, worries of the day, and all external negative influences. Relaxation at its finest, most blissful, and most rewarding.

01
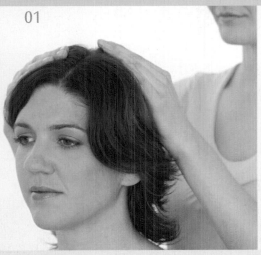

02
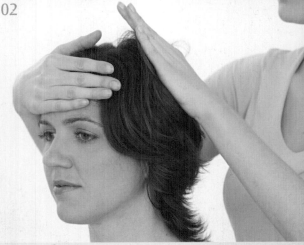

### RUBBING

*This movement is light and invigorating, and stimulates circulation to the scalp.*

*(01) Stand behind your partner and place your hands on either side of the head. Using both hands in*

*a side-to-side movement similar to hacking, but making contact with the palms of your hands instead of the outer edges, lightly rub over the whole of your partner's head. If you prefer, you can work with one hand at a time.*

*(02) Support your partner's forehead with one hand and with the palm of the other hand rub lightly over one side of the head. Change hands and repeat over the other side of the head. Make sure you cover the whole of the head with this stroke.*

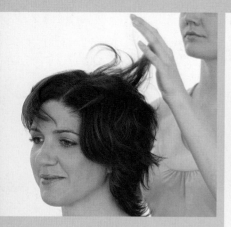

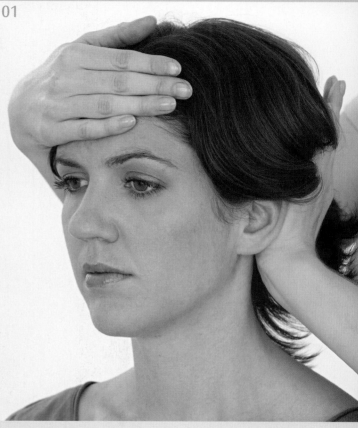

01

### LIGHT HAIR LIFTING

*This movement releases any trapped energy within the hair and makes the receiver feel very light, almost as if they are floating.*

*Starting at the back of your partner's head and working forwards, lightly run your fingers into and up through the hair in swift, flicking movements. Cover the whole of the head with this stroke.*
*If your partner has very short hair, or none at all, you can still do this stroke by using your fingertips and flicking all over the head as if the hair were there. This will release and energize the scalp in the same way.*

### MOVING THE SCALP

*This routine will help to relax and free up the scalp, and improve the flow of nutrients to the hair.*

*(01) Support your partner's forehead with one hand. Press the palm of your other hand on the back of the head, just behind the ear. By holding your position on the scalp and moving your hand in small rotations, you can force the scalp to move slightly in circles.*

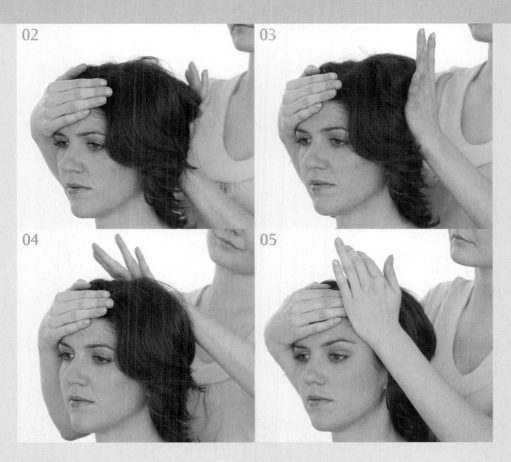

(02) Move your hand towards the back of the head by 8 cm (3¼ in) and repeat.

(03) Place your hand just above your partner's ear and repeat.

(04) Staying at the same level, move your hand towards the back of the head by 8 cm (3¼ in) and repeat.

(05) Place your hand on the top of your partner's head above the temple and repeat.

Now change hands and work all over the other side of the head, from the back to the front.

### TAPPING AND HACKING
*Use a relaxed hand when tapping so that your fingers bounce off your partner's head, and a firm, rigid hand when hacking to stimulate blood flow to the brain. You may have to change your position as you work around the sides of the head.*

*(01) Start with tapping. Curl your fingers in a loose manner and bounce one hand after the other all over your partner's head, working briskly and lightly from the front towards the back.*

*(02) Change to hacking. Hold your hands rigidly so that the strength is being transmitted to the striking edge. Again, work swiftly, one hand after the other, all over your partner's head, this time from the back towards the front. The strike should be firm but not too heavy.*

01

02

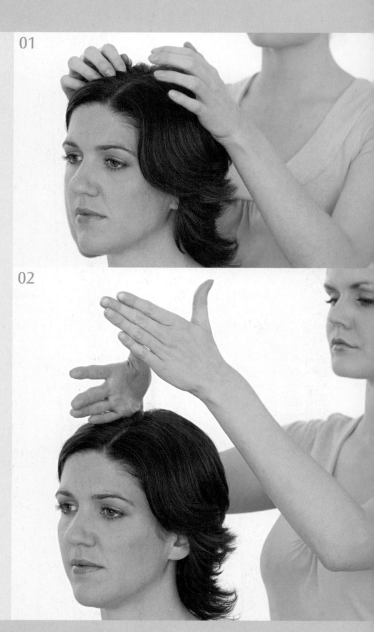

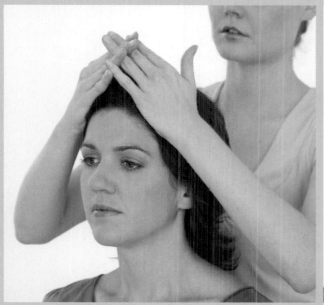 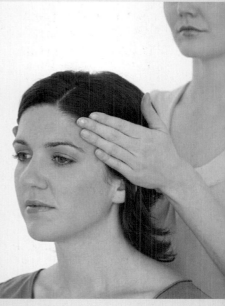

### HEAD SQUEEZING

*Tension headaches respond quickly to this technique.*

*Place the heels of your hands on your partner's temples and interlock your fingers. Squeeze inwards while at the same time pushing the heels of your hands in an upwards direction. Slide your hands upwards and release. Move your hands back towards you by about 5 cm (2 in) and repeat the technique.*

*Move your hands back to just behind your partner's ears and repeat the technique twice in this position.*

*Move your hands forwards away from you by about 5 cm (2 in) and repeat.*

*Move your hands forwards again to just over the temples and repeat once more.*

### HOLDING

*This is a very calming move, which also signals the close of the head massage and prepares your partner for the start of the face massage.*

*Place your hands on either side of your partner's head to offer light support and hold for three to five breaths.*

## FACE WORK

Working on the face helps to tone and relax the facial muscles, reduce wrinkles, and remove excess deposits of fat, toxins, oils, and dead cells from the facial area. Always work in an upwards direction, away from the pull of gravity.

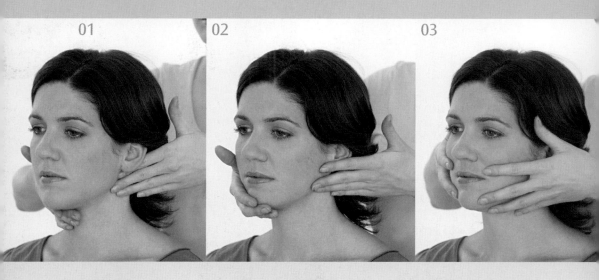

01   02   03

### STROKING

This is a very light, calming movement which can be used in order to accustom the facial muscles to being touched.

(01) Place your fingertips in a vertical line on either side of the centre of your partner's throat. Stroke lightly and gently, drawing each hand back and up towards the ears in turn. Repeat four to five times.

(02) Place your fingertips just under the chin and stroke back towards the ears. Repeat four to five times.

(03) With your index fingers meeting under your partner's nose and the other fingers meeting under the chin, stroke back towards the ears four to five times.

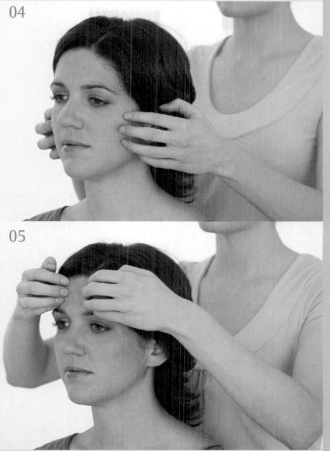

04

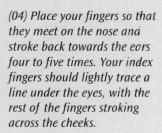

05

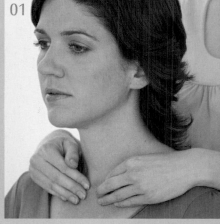

01

## LIGHT FRICTION

*This stroke helps to release any dead surface cells and stimulates circulation in the skin. The work around the nose helps to move any stagnant build-up of fluid and tissue in the nose itself, as well as in the cartilage and skin that form its shape. Use only gentle pressure while working with friction over the face and throat.*

*(04) Place your fingers so that they meet on the nose and stroke back towards the ears four to five times. Your index fingers should lightly trace a line under the eyes, with the rest of the fingers stroking across the cheeks.*

*(05) Place your fingertips together in a vertical line down the centre of your partner's forehead and stroke backwards towards the temples four to five times.*

*(01) Place your fingertips so that they meet in a vertical line at the base of your partner's throat. Lightly circle your fingers for a few moments in this position, then stroke backwards and upwards towards the ears. Repeat the stroking twice more.*

02

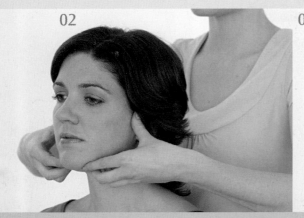

03

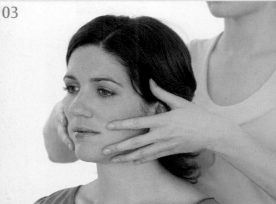

04

05

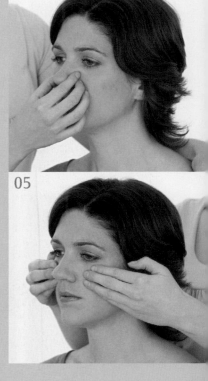

*(02) Place your thumbs on either side of your partner's face just where the upper and lower jaws meet. Hook your fingers under the lower jaw. Rotate your fingers and thumbs lightly for a few moments. Stroke lightly twice, back towards the ears. Take care not to exert too much pressure under the jaw as this could make your partner feel slightly 'strangled' and uncomfortable.*

*(03) With your index fingers meeting under your partner's nose and middle fingers meeting under the mouth, rotate in small circles. Stroke twice, back towards the ears. Move your fingers back towards the ears by about 5 cm (2 in) and repeat.*

*Continue moving your fingers back at 5 cm (2 in) intervals, repeating until you reach the ears.*

*(04) Place the fingers and thumb of one hand on either side of your partner's nose. Lightly squeeze and rotate in an upwards direction. Work up the nose in this way until you reach the bridge. Stroke twice down the nose.*

*(05) Place your index fingers on either side of your partner's nose, on the cheekbone. Position the rest of your fingers in a vertical line on the face. Rotate the fingers lightly. **Do not use this technique if your partner has had sinus drainage surgery**.*

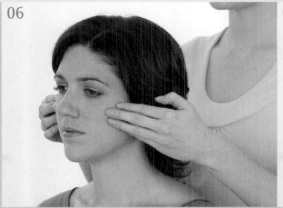

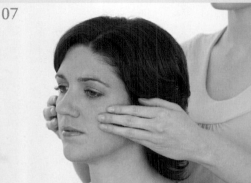

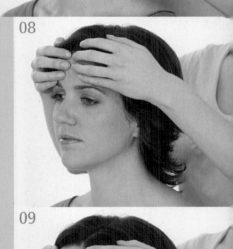

(06) Move your fingers back towards the ears by about 5 cm (2 in) and repeat.

(07) When you reach the ears, return to the first position by the nose and stroke twice backwards and upwards.

(08) Place your fingertips so that they meet in a vertical line in the middle of your partner's forehead. Apply circular rotations for a few moments. Move your fingers out by about 5 cm (2 in) and repeat the technique.

(09) Continue moving your fingers out at 5 cm (2 in) intervals, repeating the rotations at each position. When you reach your partner's temples, return to the centre of the forehead and stroke twice outwards and backwards.

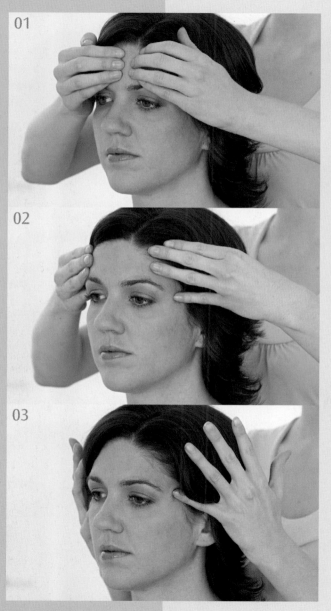

### PRESSURE

*This routine rebalances energy within the head and stimulates areas of the face that have specific effects. For example, working over the temples stimulates hormonal release within the pineal gland and calms and relaxes the mind, while applying pressure along the eyebrows relieves eyestrain and frontal headaches. When using these techniques, take care not to drag the skin downwards.*

*(01) Place the fingertips of both hands so that they meet in a vertical line in the centre of your partner's forehead. Press and hold for a count of five. Release.*

*(02) Move your fingertips apart by about 3 cm (1¼ in) and repeat. Move your fingertips apart by another 3 cm (1¼ in) and repeat. Your little fingers should now be over the temples.*

*(03) Rotate the tips of your little fingers over your partner's temples for a few moments. Release and relax.*

*(04) Using your index fingers and thumbs, pinch the innermost points on your partner's eyebrows – curled fingers below and thumbs above. Hold the pinch for a count of five.*

*(05) Move your fingers outwards by about 2 cm (¾ in) and repeat the pinch. Move your fingers outwards by another 2 cm (¾ in) and repeat. If you haven't reached the ends of your partner's eyebrows, repeat once more.*

*(06) Place your fingers in line along your partner's cheekbones. Press with a medium firmness along the cheekbones for a count of five. This stimulates and helps to drain the sinuses. Move your fingers down the face so that they hook under the cheekbones and press again for a count of five.*

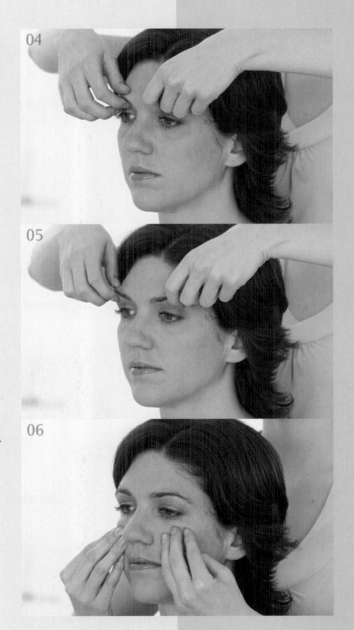

04

05

06

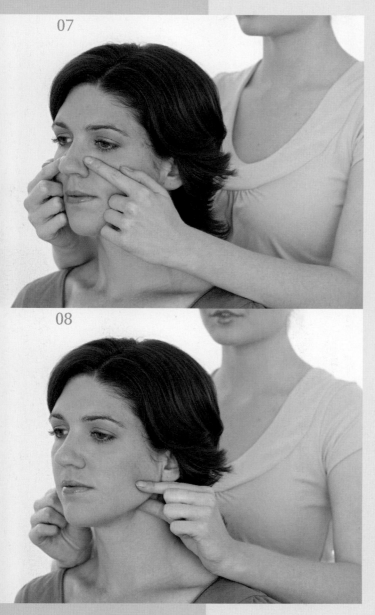

(07) Hold your index fingers on either side of the nose and rotate with a firm pressure. **Do not place any pressure on the cheekbones if your partner has had sinus drainage surgery**.

(08) Pinch all along the jawline, working from ears to chin, with a firm pressure.

To relax your partner's face after this strong work, repeat the stroking technique on pages 130–131.

## EAR MASSAGE

*If you imagine the ear as representing an upturned human body, with the lobe being the head, the outer edge the spine, and all over the inner area representing the inside of the body where the organs are situated, then you will have some idea of how each area relates to the reflexes of different parts of the body. These can be stimulated by pressure and massage to tone up your whole being. In this routine, use both hands to massage both ears at the same time.*

*(01) Start at the top of your partner's ears by pinching and rubbing them between your fingers and thumbs. Continue the pinching and rubbing all around the edge of the ears.*

*(02) When you reach the lobes, grasp and pull in a downwards direction for a few moments. Release.*

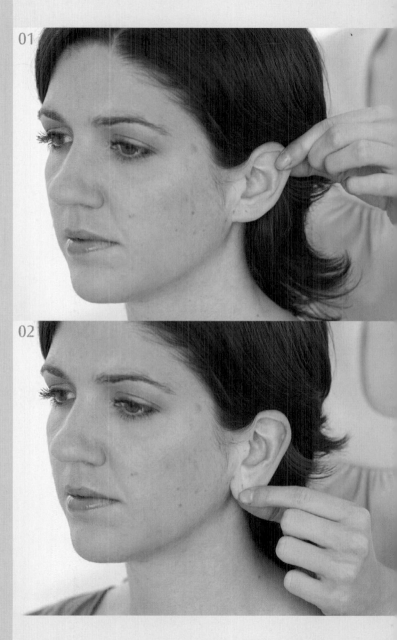

01

02

*(03) Return to the top of the ears and with the nails of your index fingers press firmly into the point where the top ridge meets the ear. Hold this position for a few moments. Release.*

*(04) Press firmly with your index fingernails under the ridge. Work along it at 1 cm (½ in) intervals, pressing firmly at each position. Continue following the ridge down to the lobes and again pull them in a downwards direction for a few moments.*

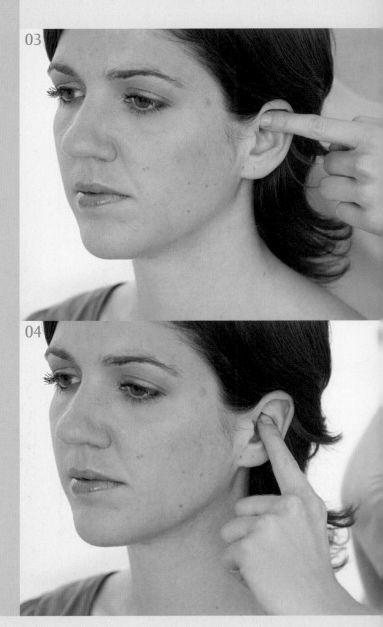

(05) Place the palms of your hands over your partner's ears and rub firmly in a rotating movement.

(06) Keeping your palms in the same position, hold in a relaxed manner while visualizing a calming light penetrating your partner's ears, then along all the nerves and fibres to the centre back of the head. Hold this position for a few moments. Release.

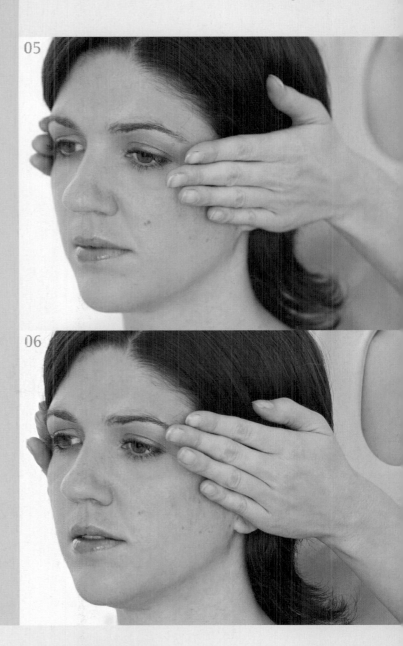

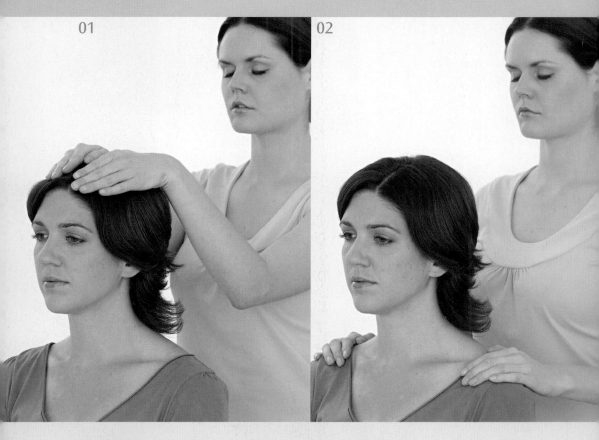

**01**

**02**

### DISCONNECTING FROM YOUR PARTNER

The connection with your partner will dissipate naturally after a few hours. However, if you wish actively to make the disconnection with your partner you can follow this procedure.

(01) Place your hands gently on your partner's head. Imagine a clear white light passing through you, into your partner, and down into the earth.

(02) Move your hands down to your partner's shoulders and continue with the visualization. Hold this position until you feel that the light has fully drained into the earth and you are both at peace. Slowly remove your hands.

# Further reading

Bentley, Eilean
*Step-by-Step Head Massage*
Gaia Books, 2000

Brennan, Barbara Ann
*Hands of Light: A Guide to Healing Through the Human Energy Field*
Bantam New Age Books, 1988

Frantzis, B. K.
*Opening the Gates of Your Body*
North Atlantic Books, 1993

Kumar, Kush
*Authentic Indian Head Massage*
Corpus Publishing, 2002

Mojay, Gabriel
*Aromatherapy for Healing the Spirit*
Gaia Books, 2005

Simpson, Liz
*The Book of Chakra Healing*
Gaia Books, 1999

# Index

skin
    broken 14
    inflamed 14, 15
    test 15, 87
slapping 66, 73
sleep 90
sliding 19, 31
squeezing 30, 33, 48, 76–7
    gentle 95–7
    head 129
    two-hand squeeze 120
squeezing and pressing 76–7
squeezing and pulling 33
stress 6, 10, 11, 37, 51, 76,
    112, 125
stroking 19, 21, 94, 122,
    130–31
stronger techniques 19

subconscious mind 8
surgery sites 62, 132
sweeping 43, 52

**T**
tapping 19, 26, 62–3, 73, 78,
    117, 128
tension 6–7, 8, 15, 21, 23, 26,
    27, 30, 32, 34, 35, 51,
    55, 56, 57, 60, 62, 64,
    68, 71, 72, 76, 78, 79,
    81, 95, 102, 113, 120,
    125
thumb pressure 113–14
thumb sliding 27
tiredness 6, 13, 15, 37, 70
touch therapies 8
toxins 7, 13, 15, 19, 30, 33, 36,

    48, 49, 72, 79, 95, 123
travelling 54–67
two-hand squeeze 120

**V**
ventilation 108
visualization 6, 10, 11, 12, 23,
    36, 38, 43, 56, 70, 85
    aura-cleansing 90–91
    cooling 83
    and intention 40–41
    waterfall 111

**W**
wake-up massages 48–9
wake-up stretches 44–7
wrinkles 130

## ACKNOWLEDGEMENTS

Editor **Leanne Bryan**
Executive Editor **Jo Godfreywood**
Executive Art Editor **Leigh Jones**
Designer **Lisa Tai**

Production Controller **Simone Nauerth**
Photographer **Ruth Jenkinson**
Models **Charlotte Medlicott** and **Victoria Barnes**
Hair and make up **Victoria Barnes**

## PICTURE CREDITS
**Special photography** © Octopus Publishing Group Limited/Ruth Jenkinson